Geriatrics

Editor

STEVEN D. JOHNSON

PHYSICIAN ASSISTANT CLINICS

www.physicianassistant.theclinics.com

Consulting Editor
JAMES A. VAN RHEE

October 2018 • Volume 3 • Number 4

ELSEVIER

1600 John F. Kennedy Boulevard • Suite 1800 • Philadelphia, Pennsylvania, 19103-2899

http://www.theclinics.com

PHYSICIAN ASSISTANT CLINICS Volume 3, Number 4
October 2018 ISSN 2405-7991, ISBN-13: 978-0-323-64114-2

Editor: Jessica McCool
Developmental Editor: Casey Potter

Physician Assistant Clinics (ISSN: 2405–7991) is published quarterly by Elsevier Inc., 360 Park Avenue South, New York, NY 10010-1710. Months of issue are January, April, July, and October. Periodicals postage paid at New York, NY and additional mailing offices. Subscription prices are $150.00 per year (US individuals), $205.00 (US institutions), $100.00 (US students), $150.00 (Canadian individuals), $257.00 (Canadian institutions), $100.00 (Canadian students), $150.00 (international individuals), $257.00 (international institutions), and $100.00 (international students). Foreign air speed delivery is included in all *Clinics* subscription prices. All prices are subject to change without notice. POSTMASTER: Send address changes to *Physician Assistant Clinics*, Elsevier Periodicals Customer Service, 11830 Westline Industrial Drive, St. Louis, MO 63146. Customer Service Health Sciences Division, Subscription Customer Service, 3251 Riverport Lane, Maryland Heights, MO 63043. **Customer Service: 1-800-654-2452 (U.S. and Canada); 314-447-8871 (outside U.S. and Canada). Fax: 314-447-8029. E-mail: journalscustomerservice-usa@elsevier.com (for print support); journalsonlinesupport-usa@elsevier.com (for online support).**

Reprints. For copies of 100 or more, of articles in this publication, please contact the Commercial Reprints Department, Elsevier Inc., 360 Park Avenue South, New York, NY 10010-1710. Tel. 212-633-3874; Fax: 212-633-3820; E-mail: reprints@elsevier.com.

Physician Assistant Clinics is covered in *EMBASE/Excerpta Medica and ESCI*.

PROGRAM OBJECTIVE
The goal of the *Physician Assistant Clinics* is to keep practicing physician assistants up to date with current clinical practice by providing timely articles reviewing the state of the art in patient care.

TARGET AUDIENCE
Physician Assistants and other healthcare professionals.

LEARNING OBJECTIVES
Upon completion of this activity, participants will be able to:
1. Review the importance of elder care.
2. Discuss treatment for depression in older adults.
3. Recognize when to refer during the primary care evaluation of cognitive decline and dementia.

ACCREDITATION
The Elsevier Office of Continuing Medical Education (EOCME) is accredited by the Accreditation Council for Continuing Medical Education (ACCME) to provide continuing medical education for physicians.

The EOCME designates this enduring material for a maximum of 15 *AMA PRA Category 1 Credit*(s)™. Physicians should claim only the credit commensurate with the extent of their participation in the activity.

All other health care professionals requesting continuing education credit for this enduring material will be issued a certificate of participation.

DISCLOSURE OF CONFLICTS OF INTEREST
The EOCME assesses conflict of interest with its instructors, faculty, planners, and other individuals who are in a position to control the content of CME activities. All relevant conflicts of interest that are identified are thoroughly vetted by EOCME for fair balance, scientific objectivity, and patient care recommendations. EOCME is committed to providing its learners with CME activities that promote improvements or quality in healthcare and not a specific proprietary business or a commercial interest.

The planning committee, staff, authors and editors listed below have identified no financial relationships or relationships to products or devices they or their spouse/life partner have with commercial interest related to the content of this CME activity:
Richard J. Ackermann, MD; Demetra Antimisiaris, PharmD, BCGP, FASCP; Walter M. Bortz II, MD; David A. Casey, MD; Lisa Cocco, MMS, PA-C; Timothy Cutler, PharmD, BCGP; Joseph Daniel; Rosegenee Ellis, MD; Casey Jackson; Steven D. Johnson, PA-C; Kathy Kemle, MS, PA-C, DFAAPA; Alison Kemp; Susan D. Leonard, MD; Jessica McCool; Dipesh Patel, MD; Kelley Queale, BA; Freddi Segal-Gidan, PA, PhD; Judy Thomas, JD; Hong-Phuc T. Tran, MD; Amy Vandenbroucke, JD, James A. Van Rhee, MS, PA-C.

UNAPPROVED/OFF-LABEL USE DISCLOSURE
The EOCME requires CME faculty to disclose to the participants:
1. When products or procedures being discussed are off-label, unlabelled, experimental, and/or investigational (not US Food and Drug Administration [FDA] approved); and
2. Any limitations on the information presented, such as data that are preliminary or that represent ongoing research, interim analyses, and/or unsupported opinions. Faculty may discuss information about pharmaceutical agents that is outside of FDA-approved labelling. This information is intended solely for CME and is not intended to promote off-label use of these medications. If you have any questions, contact the medical affairs department of the manufacturer for the most recent prescribing information.

TO ENROLL
The CME program is available to all *Physician Assistant Clinics* subscribers at no additional fee. To subscribe to the *Physician Assistant Clinics*, call customer service at 1-800-654-2452 or sign up online at www.physicianassistant.theclinics.com.

METHOD OF PARTICIPATION
In order to claim credit, participants must complete the following:
1. Complete enrolment as indicated above.
2. Read the activity.

3. Complete the CME Test and Evaluation. Participants must achieve a score of 70% on the test. All CME Tests and Evaluations must be completed online.

CME INQUIRIES/SPECIAL NEEDS
For all CME inquiries or special needs, please contact elsevierCME@elsevier.com.

Contributors

CONSULTING EDITOR

JAMES A. VAN RHEE, MS, PA-C
Associate Professor, Program Director, Yale School of Medicine, Yale Physician Assistant Online Program, New Haven, Connecticut

EDITOR

STEVEN D. JOHNSON, PA-C
Primary Care Associate Certificate, Stanford University/Foothill Community College, Stanford, California; Sutter Health, Palo Alto Medical Foundation, Palo Alto Division, The Guzik Family Center for Geriatrics and Palliative Care, Palo Alto, California; American Academy of Physician Assistants, Society of Physician Assistants Caring for the Elderly, President, Alexandria, Virginia

AUTHORS

RICHARD J. ACKERMANN, MD
Director, Hospice and Palliative Medicine Fellowship, Medical Center Navicent Health, Professor of Family Medicine, Mercer University School of Medicine, Macon, Georgia

DEMETRA ANTIMISIARIS, PharmD, BCGP, FASCP
Director, Polypharmacy and Medication Management Program, Associate Professor, Departments of Pharmacology and Toxicology, Neurology, and Family and Geriatric Medicine, University of Louisville School of Medicine, Louisville, Kentucky

WALTER M. BORTZ II, MD
Clinical Professor, Medicine Stanford University, Portola Valley, California

DAVID A. CASEY, MD
Chief of the Geriatric Psychiatry Program, Professor and Chair, Department of Psychiatry and Behavioral Sciences, University of Louisville School of Medicine, Louisville, Kentucky

LISA COCCO, MMS, PA-C
Pain Management, Internal Medicine

TIMOTHY CUTLER, PharmD, BCGP
Professor, Department of Clinical Pharmacy, University of California, San Francisco School of Pharmacy, San Francisco, California

ROSEGENEE ELLIS, MD
Medical Director, Palliative Care Service, Medical Center Navicent Health, Macon, Georgia

STEVEN D. JOHNSON, PA-C
Primary Care Associate Certificate, Stanford University/Foothill Community College, Stanford, California; Sutter Health, Palo Alto Medical Foundation, Palo Alto Division, The Guzik Family Center for Geriatrics and Palliative Care, Palo Alto, California; American Academy of Physician Assistants, Society of Physician Assistants Caring for the Elderly, President, Alexandria, Virginia

KATHY KEMLE, MS, PA-C, DFAAPA
Assistant Professor, Division of Geriatrics, Department of Family Medicine, Medical Center of Central Georgia, Navicent Health, Family Health Center, Macon, Georgia

SUSAN D. LEONARD, MD
Assistant Clinical Professor, Division of Geriatrics, University of California, Los Angeles, Los Angeles, California

DIPESH PATEL, MD
Assistant Professor, Division of Geriatrics, Department of Family Medicine, Medical Center of Central Georgia, Navicent Health, Family Health Center, Macon, Georgia

KELLEY QUEALE, BA
Coalition for Compassionate Care of California, Sacramento, California

FREDDI SEGAL-GIDAN, PA, PhD
Keck School of Medicine of USC, University of Southern California, Rancho Los Amigos National Rehabilitation Center, Rancho/USC California Alzheimers Disease Center, Downey, California

JUDY THOMAS, JD
Coalition for Compassionate Care of California, Sacramento, California

HONG-PHUC T. TRAN, MD
Assistant Clinical Professor, Division of Geriatrics, University of California, Los Angeles, Los Angeles, California

AMY VANDENBROUCKE, JD
National POLST Paradigm, Washington, DC

Contents

The United States is experiencing a significant population shift with the aging of the baby boomers. The silver tsunami combined with the projected decrease of the physician workforce and geriatric physicians will significantly affect primary care. It is reasonable to assume that physician assistants will assume greater responsibility for the clinical and social management of increasing numbers of frail, medically complex, older adults. These trends will significantly challenge primary care clinic schedules and, possibly, the location where medical care is provided.

As the population ages, falls among older adults are a growing public health concern. Because they are multifactorial, a multipronged approach involving a team is needed to address them. Physician assistants are essential providers in emergency rooms, hospitals, nursing homes, and outpatient areas and can play a vital role in screening and intervention to reduce risk. Older adults should be screened for risk factors associated with falls, and these should be addressed. Exercise programs, vitamin D supplementation, reduction of unnecessary and harmful medications, correction of visual impairment, and environmental modification hold the greatest promise for decreasing falls and related injuries.

Cognitive decline becomes increasingly common with advanced age. Early signs and symptoms may be subtle and overlooked by patients and family members and missed or discounted by providers. Screening offers an opportunity for early detection, providing multiple benefits. For patients who screen positive or with complaints of memory loss or other cognitive changes, evaluation is required to identify contributing or reversible causes. Screening and detection tools that are easy to access and use are discussed. Diagnosis can be made through a basic primary care evaluation, but some cases may require referral to specialist.

This article is an overview of advance care planning, which is a process that supports adults at any age or stage of health understand and share their personal values, life goals, and preferences regarding future medical care. It increases the likelihood that an individual's treatment wishes will be known and respected during serious illness and at the end of life. Advance directives and physician orders for life-sustaining treatment are defined, compared, and contrasted.

Palliative care should be part of the expertise of physician assistants caring for older adults. Palliative care is an integrated, holistic approach to patients with severe and terminal illness, whereas hospice is a defined benefit for patients with a life expectancy shorter than 6 months. If an older adult lacks decision-making capacity, a family member needs to act as surrogate. That person should use the principle of substituted judgment, advocating for what the patient would decide in that situation.

The incidence of chronic pain in the functional geriatric adult is high, and there is an outcry among providers for fast and objective methods to manage pain and preserve functional capacity in this population. The purpose of this article is to acquaint providers with evidence-based tools and pearls of wisdom for practice that are easy to administer, that can be applied to all patients as part of a foundational screening or as needed when clinically indicated, and that establish clear goals and accountability in the management of pain as a symptom of disability.

Depression is not a normal part of the aging process. Depression in older adults is a treatable medical condition; a variety of psychotherapeutic options are available. Electroconvulsive therapy is a useful treatment. Older patients must be viewed in their medical, functional, and social context for effective management. Cognition must be assessed along with mood in the older patient with depression.

Polypharmacy is an underappreciated factor in undesirable patient out-comes. In older adults, polypharmacy is considered a syndrome of harm and presents a challenge to primary care providers. The United States has one of the highest medication use rates per capita in the world. With the aging population, and polypharmacy a significant part of the lives of older adults, management of polypharmacy poses both a growing chal-lenge and an opportunity for all health care providers. This article provides an overview of skills to improve medication use management in older adults living with polypharmacy.

Because of a growing, aging population and a shortage of geriatricians in the United States, the care of geriatric patients will mostly devolve to pri-mary care providers. This article reviews the different aspects of a multidi-mensional, multidisciplinary geriatric assessment. Assessment tools and training of office staff to take on larger roles can help primary care pro-viders reduce the burden of work associated with performing a compre-hensive geriatric assessment.

PHYSICIAN ASSISTANT CLINICS

FORTHCOMING ISSUES

January 2019
Primary Care of the Medically Underserved
Vincent Morelli, Roger Zoorab,
and Joel J. Heidelbaugh, *Editors*

April 2019
Critical Care Medicine
Kim Zuber and Jane S. Davis, *Editors*

July 2019
Laboratory Medicine
Jane McDaniel, *Editor*

RECENT ISSUES

July 2018
Women's Health
Heather P. Adams and
Aleece Fosnight, *Editors*

April 2018
Otolaryngology
Laura A. Kirk, *Editor*

January 2018
Urology
Todd J. Doran, *Editor*

RELATED INTEREST

Clinics in Geriatric Medicine, February 2018 (Vol. 34, Issue 1)
Screening and Prevention in Geriatric Medicine
Danelle Cayea and Samuel C. Durso, *Editors*

THE CLINICS ARE AVAILABLE ONLINE!
Access your subscription at:
www.theclinics.com

Foreword

An Aging Population

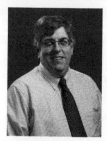

James A. Van Rhee, MS, PA-C
Consulting Editor

According to the US Census Bureau, the United States will experience considerable growth in its older population. In 2050, the population aged 65 and over is projected to be 83.7 million, almost double its estimated population of 43.2 million in 2012.[1] With this growth in the elderly population will come an increased demand for health care providers. Physician assistants can meet this need and have been shown to have a huge effect in caring for the elderly. For example, a study by Ackermann and Kemle (both have written articles for this issue) showed that regular visits to nursing home patients by a physician assistant can reduce hospitalization and medical costs for these older people.[2]

Steven Johnson, the guest editor for this issue, has put together a group of talented and knowledgeable authors to cover topics in geriatrics that are important to physician assistants in any area of clinical practice. The articles in this issue are not reviews of a variety of disease states noted in the elderly patient population, but they address the overall care of the elderly patient.

Falls are common in the geriatric population, and the evaluation and management of falls in the elderly patient is covered by Kemle. Evaluation of cognitive decline and dementia is covered by Segal-Gidan. Advanced care planning, a topic all clinicians have to deal with in all areas of practice, is covered by Queale, Thomas, and Vandebroucke; they provide some excellent tips and ideas on dealing with patients and their families in advanced care planning. Palliative care is covered by Ackerman, and the functional assessment and management of pain is reviewed by Cocco. Two very common issues, depression in the elderly, covered by Casey, and polypharmacy, covered by Antimisiaris and Cutler, are addressed. I also want to highlight the articles on successful aging by Bortz and geriatric assessment by Tran and Leonard; these provide an excellent overview of the normal aging and general assessment of the geriatric patient.

Physician Assist Clin 3 (2018) xi–xii
https://doi.org/10.1016/j.cpha.2018.07.002
2405-7991/18/© 2018 Published by Elsevier Inc.

This issue provides you with a wealth of new information on the care of the elderly patient that you can utilize every day in your practice. Our next issue will provide you with a review of the latest in laboratory medicine.

James A. Van Rhee, MS, PA-C
Yale School of Medicine
Yale Physician Assistant Online Program
100 Church Street South, Suite A230
New Haven, CT 06519, USA

E-mail address:
james.vanrhee@yale.edu

Website:
http://www.paonline.yale.edu

REFERENCES

1. Ortman JM, Velkoff VA, Hogan H. An aging nation: the older population in the United States, current population reports. Washington, DC: US Census Bureau; 2014. p. 25–1140.
2. Ackermann RJ, Kemle KA. The effect of a physician assistant on the hospitalization of nursing home residents. J Am Geriatr Soc 1998;46:610–4.

Preface

A Geriatric Imperative

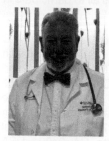

Steven D. Johnson, PA-C
Editor

There are a number of phrases used to describe the expected demographic shift where the number of adults over 65 is expected to double in the next 20 years. The Grey Tide, Silver Tsunami, an Age Wave, and the Grey Hoard are a few. It is reasonable to expect that with our aging population there will be a significant day-to-day impact on society and health care, and especially, primary care medicine. While all specialties will be tasked with older patients, I believe that primary care will be stressed with the management of the frail older adult and the associated family, social, community, and medical challenges that are inevitably part of geriatric care. This shift creates a very real health care and social Geriatric Imperative: not a descriptor but a call to action.

The Geriatric Imperative requires that we support and create teams of skilled providers across specialties and professions to assess and manage older adults. The Geriatric Imperative requires time to assess, treat, explore family and social support, and coordinate elder care. The Geriatric Imperative requires federal, state, county, city, and community funding and support for community social support networks, senior centers, transportation, home health services. The Geriatric Imperative will require loosening of restrictive regulations that impair well-trained professionals from functioning in a team environment from the office, home, hospital, and nursing facility. The Geriatric Imperative will require multiple professionals (physicians, physical and occupational therapists, social workers, nursing, nurse practitioners, and physician assistants [PA]) to schedule time for counseling patient and family. The Geriatric Imperative will require employer accommodation for employees faced with the challenges of caring for children and aging parents. The Geriatric Imperative will demand new patient and family–centered innovations for place of care and bedside clinical diagnostics. And, finally, the Geriatric Imperative requires that we strongly advocate for payment mechanisms that recognize the demands of frail elder care and adequately compensate the provider for this time-intensive work.

Physician Assist Clin 3 (2018) xiii–xiv
https://doi.org/10.1016/j.cpha.2018.07.001
2405-7991/18/© 2018 Published by Elsevier Inc.

physicianassistant.theclinics.com

In this issue of *Physician Assistant Clinics*, we have created a primer on many of the social and clinical challenges we are and will be facing with an aging population. I am deeply indebted to the extraordinary physicians, pharmacists, and PAs who have contributed to this issue. I hope that this issue will serve as a resource for you as we all prepare for the challenges of caring and accommodating an aging population. I also hope that this issue will serve as a PA call to action and for us all to participate in the Geriatric Imperative.

Steven D. Johnson, PA-C
Sutter Health
Palo Alto Medical Foundation
Guzik Family Center for Geriatrics
and Palliative Care
Geriatric Medicine Team
795 El Camino Real
Palo Alto, CA, 94301, USA

E-mail address:
johnsot5@sutterhealth.org

Erratum

The forthcoming issues page in the July 2018 issue of *Physician Assistant Clinics* (Volume 3, Issue 3) incorrectly listed the upcoming January 2019 issue as "Laboratory Medicine" edited by Jane McDaniel. This issue will be the July 2019 issue. The January 2019 issue will be "Primary Care of the Medically Underserved" edited by Drs. Vincent Morelli, Roger Zoorab, and Joel J. Heidelbaugh.

Physician Assist Clin 3 (2018) xv
https://doi.org/10.1016/j.cpha.2018.07.004
2405-7991/18/© 2018 Published by Elsevier Inc.

physicianassistant.theclinics.com

Erratum

The forthcoming issues page in the July 2018 issue of Physician Assistant Clinics (volume 3, issue 3) incorrectly listed the upcoming January 2019 issue as "Laboratory Medicine," edited by Jane McDaniel. This issue will be the July 2019 issue. The January 2019 issue will be "Primary Care of the Medically Underserved," edited by Drs. Vincent Morelli, Roger Zoorob, and Joel J. Heidelbaugh, Jr.

Editorial
Physician Assistants, Geriatrics, and Next Medicine

Before birth, medicine was in my umbilical blood. I am a doctor (MD), University of Pennsylvania, 1955. My father was a doctor (MD), Harvard, 1921. I was named for a doctor (MD), Jefferson, 1910. I married the daughter of a doctor (MD), Tufts, 1928. I am the father of a doctor (MD), Boston University, 1992. I am grandfather to an RN, Oregon Health Sciences, 2015. I am the cousin of a doctor (MD), Jefferson, 1951.

My medical resume overflows. Certainly, this genealogy was a major contributor to the discomfort that troubled me so deeply in 2011 when I wrote my magnus opus, *Next Medicine, the Science and Civics of Health*, for Oxford University Press.[1] I dedicated the book to the "renaissance of my profession." It received strong reviews in *Science*, *Journal of the American Medical Association*, and the *Wall Street Journal*. I continue to lecture on its precepts that represent a wide-ranging critique of my profession that dad called "a jealous mistress." I have embraced Oliver Holmes' urging: "If you would go off like an opium eater in love with your starving delusions, be a doctor." My idealism is strained. Steve Schroeder asked, "Has Medicine lost its soul?"

In my book, I listed medicines, symptoms which are very costly, inequity, harmfulness, inefficiency, corruption, but most egregious of all, irrelevance.

If a patient enters my office with a similar set of complaints, I will inevitably conclude that the only possible diagnosis is total body pain, a too common condition that does not lend itself to reductionist analysis. No single cell or organ or process is responsible. Rather, it is the whole system that aches. Despite huge gains in technical advances and grotesque gains in financial commitment, medicine is generally regarded as derelict in fulfilling its job description. We are forced to ask, just what *is* medicine's job?

This prompts a search for guiding principles. Thomas Kuhn's[2] 1962 magisterial book, entitled *The Structure of Scientific Revolutions*, is vitally helpful. His book concludes that in order for a satisfactory outcome to an intolerable challenge to occur, two prerequisites must be met. These are, first, agreement among all the aggrieved parties that a revolution must occur. The second, and more critical precondition, is the availability of a replacement paradigm. This connotes that a sturdy administrative structure be available to replace the defective one.

Kuhn utilizes the challenges faced by the colonists in 1770 as his case statement. On July 4, 1776, all 13 colonies signed on to our Declaration of Independence, and the requisite unanimity of commitment was fulfilled. The second prerequisite remained to be addressed. After a few years, representatives from the 13 colonies met again in Philadelphia and produced a replacement paradigm that became the Constitution of the United States of America. Democracy rather than Monarchy was the new paradigm. The two prerequisites were fulfilled, and we became a nation, a scientific revolution assured by Kuhn's formula.

In my book, I invoked Kuhn's process for Medicine's troubled present. There is certainly near consensus that the scene is set for a revolution. Democrats and

Physician Assist Clin 3 (2018) xvii–xxv
https://doi.org/10.1016/j.cpha.2018.05.010
2405-7991/18/© 2018 Published by Elsevier Inc.

Republicans, east, south, north, and west, Labor and Industry, young and old all maneuver for a replacement paradigm. So this consensus is at hand. What remains is the provision of an adequate replacement paradigm for the defective administrative apparatus currently in place.

SEEKING MISSION

In my view, current Medicine is in the disease business; it should be in the health business. Its entire enterprise is directed to repair. Its tools are drugs, surgery, and techniques, all predicated on treating a problem, on curing. Instead, incentives should fixate on the preservation of well-being. Health rather than disease should be the new paradigm.

The issue of structural lag is important here.[3] This fact promulgated by John and Matilda Riley observes that society displays a substantial lag between the occurrence of a problem and its societal response. Wars and financial crises are common examples. Our present medical system was derived from the era of catastrophic illnesses mostly infectious in origin. Survival even until middle age was a rarity. Smallpox, cholera, and their evil compatriots raged the globe. Medical Science was inert. Not until Pasteur rescued the globe did panic ease. Sanitation and antisepsis birthed modern surgery. Antibiotics, anesthesia, and insulin changed the world. Modern medicine emerged.

That was then. This is now. An entirely new array of health challenges emerges.[4] Instead of acute episodic illnesses being dominant, we are confronted with an epidemic of chronic diseases with diffuse origins. We are in a structural lag with outdated philosophies and strategies. We confront problems with a curative mindset, while our current challenges are not curable. But they are preventable.

Zimmerman's Law states no one notices when things go right. This simple homily underlies the fact 95% of the US health care economy is allocated to direct medical treatment with a curative hope. Less than 5% is allocated to health improvement. Medical science has dedicated almost the entirety of its intellectual and financial capital to disease treatment. I am reminded of one of Victor Borge's skits that portrays his uncle, who became severely depressed because he discovered a treatment for which there was no disease. Our health care system is really our disease care system. Our health insurance is really disease insurance. The National Institutes of Health is really the National Institutes of Disease. Our emphasis is on panacea not on hygeia.

Not only is our medical system rigged to confront illness at the practice level but also this perspective extends to medical education and workforce. The classroom for medical students and trainees is the hospital and, particularly, the intensive care unit. This is where the glamour and the payment mechanisms prevail. Medical subspecialty and sub-subspecialty is the game plan. Most illness however does not conform to this design. Clayton Christensen,[5] esteemed professor at Harvard Business School, is the principal advocate for disruptive innovation, for revolution. His book, *Disruptive Prescription*, elaborately details how the infrastructure of current medicine is ill suited to its task. He notes with approval the development of nontraditional medical care sites such as pharmacies and supermarkets. He is a strenuous advocate for lesser medical expertise within the curriculum of medical schools. I and most of us medics are far overtrained for day-to-day clinical tasks. I am very proud of Stanford University School of Medicine, my home church, which has pursued the training of Physician Assistants by including a PA master's degree program in its catalog. In my busy practice as a geriatrician, I have found it critical to associate with a non–physician practitioner to deliver adequate care. A Physician Assistant is my personal primary care provider. I honor them categorically.

With leadership from my friend Eddie Phillips at Harvard, we have initiated a new course within the medical school on behavioral medicine. We identified that diet and exercise and sleep and meditation were missing from the standard curriculum. Consequently, for four years, we have provided such training within the medical school, but also with attendance from other parts of the campus.

I would lobby for a greatly expanded health emphasis in grade school and early education. I have worked with the local department of education to insert health promotion into their efforts. I take greatest delight in lecturing second-grade students on the perils of diabetes, a huge disease challenge that Current Medicine seems impotent to confront. I hope the kids take my prevention messages home at night.

The Internet presents Next Medicine with immense opportunities for self-care. My friendship with Albert Bandura, premier psychologist here at Stanford, leads me to conclude that self-efficacy is a central feature of health preservation.[6] Mobilization of the "healer within" requires every opportunity to do its magic. Bandura writes a prescription for self-efficacy much as I write one for penicillin.

The first component in building personal self-efficacy involves the setting of small steps of mastery (i.e., walk to the post office instead of driving). Second is peer examples (ie, if Sam can do it, so can you). Third is diminishment of cues of failure (ie, if your feet hurt after a jog, get bigger shoes), and last is social persuasion, which is simply the mustering of the overwhelming evidence that self-improvement is possible. Bandura rejects the perspective that you can't change human nature. He insists that you're not trying to change nature, only nurture, which is eminently more malleable.

I am convinced that health illiteracy kills more people than disease, and it is our corporate responsibility to address health illiteracy wherever and whenever it presents. A healthy longevity correlates well with health literacy.

THE MISSION OF MEDICINE

As Medicine seeks to justify its exalted societal role, I nominate a new mission for my profession: *the assertion and assurance of the human potential*, to identify our functional and structural potential, and to pursue strategies that give best hope for attaining and retaining this. Of course, this is where my background as a geriatrician appears. It is my conviction that 100 healthy years represent the essence of the human potential.

In my view, the most important medical article published in my lifetime was by McGinnis and Foege[7] in *Journal of the American Medical Association* in 1993. The title of their article was "Actual Causes of Death in the United States."[7] Instead of the traditional heart, cancer, stroke, nomenclature, they portrayed that it is the underlying behavioral substrate that is the villain. This acknowledges the powerful social forces in play, but emphasizes that biological influences are more proximate in their causation.

DETERMINING HEALTH

Borrowing from their format, I wrote an article for the *American Journal of Public Health* in 2005 entitled, "Biological Basis of Determinants of Health."[8] I analogized that human health determinants are the same as those of an automobile, four in number: design, accidents, maintenance, and aging. Clearly, a car with fundamental structural or functional defects, a lemon, will be lucky to get off the showroom floor. If the car insists on running into other cars or over cliffs, its existence is precarious. If it is poorly maintained, it will not be on the highway very long. And finally, over time it will wear out as all things do.

Design

Most abnormal fetuses are expelled in utero as spontaneous abortions, so that virtually all newborns are perfect. Strohman estimates that less than 2% of human illness is attributable to an abnormal gene locus.[9] Virtually all diseases exhibit mosaic patterns with complexity at each step. Evolution dictates that we are gloriously designed.

Accidents

Accidents of many kinds are a clear and constant danger. Throughout history, the major threat to human health has been a by-product of an adverse encounter with a hostile threat. Pasteur demonstrated that the previously held attribution of sickness to metaphysical punishment motifs was wrong, that a microbe was more properly labeled as the devil. Another historical threat has been starvation that at different times has threatened extinction of large segments of the population. Wars have killed off millions of our species. Trauma shortens lives.

Most accidents are preventable.

Maintenance

Like a car's maintenance, ours involves fuel and rpms. Poor quality or wrong amount of fuel invites problems. Obesity is a global threat. Another determinative maintenance issue is energy flow, rpms. Racing the engine or allowing it to idle too long is precarious. Too many rpms present as stress, the systemic results of which Hans Selye[10] called the general adaptation syndrome: secondary to too heavy an allostatic load, the cumulative toll exerted on the body's structural and functional responsiveness to excessive environmental load.

The converse of stress is disuse, a physiologic state that has been of absorbing interest to me for decades, ever since my leg was in a cast after I had ruptured my Achilles tendon while skiing fifty years ago. My leg became precociously old because of the enforced inactivity. Disuse means too little energetic exchange with the environment, usually manifested through a sedentary lifestyle.

I have codified the common clinical parameters within this rubric as the disuse syndrome.[11] Its components are cardiovascular vulnerability, musculoskeletal fragility, metabolic instability, immunologic susceptibility, depression, and frailty.

AGING

Indelible is the fact that the Gray Dawn of Aging is upon us.[12] No household or country is immune to this powerful mandate. Current census data indicate that 15% of Americans are now over 65 years of old, and this is projected to more than double from 46 million today to over 60 million by 2060. The elderly population will rise to nearly 24% from the current 15%. One in four of us will be over 65.

The transformative effects of this trend are pervasive. Among the more universal are the effects that population aging will have on medical care. In 1974, Knight Steel and Frank Williams wrote an article entitled, "Geriatrics: The Fruition of the Condition."[13] Reading this article today reveals the lowly status of geriatrics within the general medical curriculum at that time. It was apparent that ageism had affected academic and political realms stigmatizing the whole reach of geriatrics. They referred to geriatrics "as a stepchild of medicine," but asserted that the extended scope of geriatrics, particularly its caring imperative, should represent the fruition rather than the stepchild relationship.

A major part of the diminished prestige of geriatric medicine resulted from the lack of a sturdy conceptual platform. Aging was a backwater of scientific pursuit.

Recent decades have generated major advances in biology. Ten years ago, Len Hayflick,[14] preeminent gerontologist, wrote "the biology of aging is no longer an unknown". He invoked a terse thermophysical explanation. Aging is now known. Our ignorance about aging stems largely from the premise that aging is a disease and thereby lends itself to a curative approach. This perspective is in turn largely driven by the hope for a profit. This was manifested by a cover story of *TIME* magazine a while back that asked, "Can Google solve death?" The immortalist movement finds a happy home site in this point of view. As long ago as Ponce De Leone, mankind has labored to find the secret of perpetual youth. Thousands of sheep testicles have been sacrificed in this hope. Charlatans abound, and rejuvenation is big business attracting hordes of the faithful to its cause. Plastic surgeons have never discovered a wrinkle that didn't require a tuck or two or ten. The quadrillion dollar cosmetic industry seeks to smudge away the evidence of decades.

In my view, the gene industry is also complicit in this regard. On scant evidence, millions of dollars and decades of scientific pursuit have sought a genetic origin for aging as though the organism had an in situ limit to longevity.

Until now, medicine has been on a fruitless search to find a genetic origin for aging. Just imagine the size of the bonanza that awaits discovery of "the aging gene." Counteractant potions could be infused into hair tonics, potency enhancers, or even baby formulas.

A central frontier for aging studies involves twins. Were aging primarily a genetic process, identical twins sharing the same DNA preprint should die simultaneously of the same condition. This is not the case. We obtained data from a cohort of identical twins at National Institutes of Health who were the male survivors of World War II.[15] When we looked at their mortality statistics, we found that the twins did not die simultaneously, but 6.8 years apart, and rarely of the same condition. A biostatistician then concludes that 15% of longevity is hereditary. It is clear therefore that *"it ain't cards you're dealt that matters so much as it is how you play the hand."* Martin has concluded that more than 6000 genes are involved in human aging.[16] It, like virtually all human ailments, is polygenic. Reductionism has reached its limits in this gene fixation.

Abandonment of the gene focus changed attention to the organism as a whole, the phenotype. Not only is the organism ordained by its genotype (genome wide association study) but also it is grandly influenced by the environment, the nature/nurture interface (environment wide association study).[17] The nexus of the organism within the environment is the appropriate platform for study. To a large extent, the organism becomes what it does, as phenotypic plasticity is a huge contributor to our well-being. "Use It or Lose It" is the common vernacular that captures the linkage between function and structure. We seek the physical origin of aging that is found in the tenets of the second law of thermodynamics. We wear out, just as everything else in the Universe does. The Second Law commands this.

DISUSE AND AGING

Much of what people commonly attribute to aging is instead due to disuse. The differentiation of these two components is critical because aging is not something that can be altered. It is rooted in cosmic law, but disuse is subject to behavioral intervention. I am a fervent student of the serenity prayer, to change what I can, but accept that which I can't. This is an optimistic perspective.

I published an article in *Journal of the American Geriatric Society* 30 years ago called "Redefining Human Aging."[18] It provides a generic formulation of the determinative health agencies of older people. Three separate and distinct mechanisms are proposed to distinguish the fundamental processes that underlie the heterogeneity of clinical patterns of old people. "A grandfather's clock stops running. Either it is worn out, it is broken, or it needs to be wound up." It is vividly clear that these three diagnostic categories, aging, disease, and disuse, are casually conflated leading to major errors and resource allocation.

A 1987 editorial in *Journal of the American Medical Association* by Wetle[19] was titled, "Age as a Risk Factor for Inadequate Treatment." Suitability for surgery, ICU admission, transplant appropriateness, dialysis, and other common circumstances exhibited an age exponential in decision making. The differential between disease, disuse, and aging is imprecise and evolving.

In the past, tuberculosis was labeled as part of the aging process. More recently, arteriosclerosis is improperly ascribed to aging. Currently, Alzheimer disease and other neurologic conditions and diabetes are often casually cited to be causes of aging processes.

Ten years ago, Hayflick[14] published a paper in the *Annals of the New York Academy of Sciences* entitled, "Biologic Aging Is no Longer an Unsolved Problem."[14] In it he promotes a definitive statement that the basis of aging is the inexorable result of thermophysical decay codified in the second law of thermodynamics that Schrodinger[20] invoked in his magisterial statement, "What is life?" This universal canon underlies all living and inanimate change. It is the source of the physical principles that govern evolution and development. Aging is the effect of an energy flow on matter over time. Hayflick makes an emphatic differentiation of disease processes from aging with which it is frequently misrepresented, resulting in confused strategies and misguided resource allocations. Such an inclusive definition of aging positions it within the organism and thereby not contingent on extrinsic agency. Aging must be differentiated from disease and disuse with which it is frequently conflated. The exclusive dominance of the disease model of medicine distorts research education and practice priorities. Like the dysfunctional grandfathers clock, all three agencies must be considered. Insistence on a categorical separation of agents and diseases is critical but insufficient. Recently, Lunney and Lynn of the Altarum Institute observed that 20% of persons die in their 60s of cancer that is miserable, costly, and painful.[21] Another 20% of people die in their 70s of a single end-organ dysfunction: heart, lung, liver, or kidney, leaving 60% still living to 80 to die of other issues. The most fragile part of the anatomy is the brain. Therefore, this conforms to the current epidemic of degenerative brain diseases that presents a whole panoply of new challenges. Some doomsayers predict that brain pathology with its assorted economic and cultural impacts will soon become the dominant threat to society. The oppressive reality of caregiver stress is huge and worthy of much more address.

Beyond this is the notion that the entirety of geropathology is distorted by insistence on a single agency. This perspective is a leftover from the infectious era that has dominated medicine for decades. We are only barely aware that emerging today is the notion of multiple accumulated assaults. There's a whole emphasis now on cumulative damage. Aging is a processing deficit accumulation. No single issue but the number of hits, much like Medawar's illustration of coffee cups, that over time damage accumulates.[22]

Personally, at age 88, my legs have given out, and my heart has remodeled and started atrial fibrillation after years of marathoning. My wife, herself a champion marathoner, wore out her hip because she had an asymmetric, ineffective gait and late in life needed a hip replacement that eventuated in her decline and demise.

A 2015 article in *Aging Cell* called, "Predicting All-Cause Mortality from Basic Physiology in the Framingham Heart Study," surveyed the standard classical risk factors for heart disease, including systolic blood pressure, blood sugar, body weight, body mass index, and cholesterol level and found that all of these markers are significant when considered at a single moment, but when they are summated and viewed over time they achieve a much higher correlation with the mortality statistics.[23] This supports the idea that it is not the individual risk factors at a given moment that are so significant as it is the cumulative hazard that all produced together.

This is a novel scientific perspective. Instead of individual risk factors or organ declines, the emphasis shifts to the organism. This translates to a categorical change in philosophy and resource allocation. We become what we do because we are plastic. When we don't, we aren't; when we don't, we are at risk. Frailty is a major component of late life. It has been the object of increasing study, led by Linda Fried, Columbia.[24] I contributed an article called, "Conceptual Framework of Frailty,"[25] and once again emphasized the role of physical activity in retarding frailty.

Medical terminology needs an update. The inadequacy of the term homeostasis popularized by Walter Cannon is derelict. Upon reflection, the term homeodynamics as proposed by Yates is much more realistic. There is no stasis in life.[26] Everything is dynamic as there's a constant interplay.

When Schrodinger[20] wrote his famous article in 1944, he bifurcated life into replication and metabolism. Replication is easily understood as the matching strands of DNA. Metabolism (from the Greek "to change") is progressively being understood by the techniques of molecular biology.

Metabolism is inherent in all life, "its 'GO'." All of this derives from the new Nanotechnology that enables visualization of physiology at the atomic level.

This illuminates the process of aging that finds complete explication as molecular decay resulting from bombardment by water molecules. This "molecular storm" shortens telomeres and generates reactive oxygen species and membrane permeability all due to this nanochaos. Peter Hoffman,[27] in his major book, "Life's Ratchet," describes that this is a reflection of the Brownian movement of water molecules that intrigued Einstein. Prigogine and Stengers[28] coined the phrase "dissipative structures" to indicate the constructive effect that energy flow causes. This bombardment of Brownian action translates into conformational changes.

These conformational changes describe the process known as symmorphosis[29] in which structure results from the summing effect of energy flow on matter over time.

We now know the intimate level of molecular interplay that happens progressively over time. Aging is not a disease. It is the inevitable by-product of entropy,[30] the Second Law of Thermodynamics in action.

CLINICAL EVIDENCE

Steve Blair and colleagues' critical paper, "Physical Exercise and All-Cause Mortality," reflects that fitness is a dominant determinant of survival and longevity, particularly after the age of 60.[31] VO_2max, our most sensitive measure of fitness, is not reflective of all-cause mortality before age 60, but becomes absolutely determinative thereafter.

The classic study of change in physical condition in 90-year-old nursing residents[32] shows that exercise can restore structural integrity even into the tenth decade.

Geriatric medicine represents a summation of the lifetime of environmental challenges. Human aging represents a natural experiment of cumulative effects of time on structure and function. Many of the late-life health syndromes are subject to active correction. Aging is a time-integrated process separate from the disease model of medicine. Rather than illness being the expression of extrinsic agents, singly or in combination, in older people it derives from the inappropriate interface of nature and nurture. Time is the essential dimension. Geriatrics is the very essence of the effect of time on structure and function. *It is never too late to start, but it's always too soon to stop.*

SUMMARY

As we seek a broad consensus for restoring America's severely dysfunctional health care system, I nominate geriatrics as an insightful text to the current mess. By definition, the Physician Assistant is poised to be a critical component of geriatric medicine. The Physician Assistant demonstrates appropriate clinical skills with a patient, family, and community focus that supports the geriatric team. The resulting model represents a replacement paradigm for Next Medicine. The art of medicine finds full display within geriatrics. Broad, not specialized, competency addresses the diffuse demands of geriatric medicine that requires a different competency and compassion. The caring aspect of geriatrics is central to its mission. Emphasis on the person as a whole rather than the component parts and on health rather than disease drives the primary focus to prevention over repair.

Rather than the ICU and laboratory being the primary workplace and logical focus of research and activity of geriatrics, it is the home, school, and office. The social world is intimate.

Geriatrics is fundamentally optimistic as it seeks the fulfillment of the human potential that is the mission of medicine. Geriatrics has its primary role the maintenance of function over time. It stresses health preservation over repair.

Old dogs and people can still learn new tricks. One hundred healthy years is our birthright. It commands each of us to assure this basic human potential.

Walter M. Bortz II, MD
Medicine Stanford University
167 Bolivar Lane
Portola Valley, CA 94028, USA

E-mail address:
drwbortz@gmail.com

REFERENCES

1. Bortz WM. Next medicine. The science and civics of health. Oxford (NY): Oxford University Press; 2011.
2. Kuhn T. The structure of scientific revolutions. Chicago: University of Chicago Press; 1962.
3. Riley M, Kahn R. Age and structural lag. Chicago: University of Chicago Press; 1962.
4. Starr P. The social transformation of American medicine. New York: Basic Books; 1986.
5. Christensen C, Raynor M. The innovator's solution. Boston: Harvard Business School Publishing; 2003.

6. Bandura A. Self-efficacy. New York: WH Freeman; 1997.
7. McGinnis JM, Foege WH. Actual causes of death in the United States. JAMA 1993;270:2207–12.
8. Bortz WM. Biological basis of determinants of health. Am J Public Health 2005; 95:389–92.
9. Strohman RC. Ancient genomes, wise bodies, unhealthy people: limits of a genetic paradigm in biology and medicine. Perspect Biol Med 1993;37:112–45.
10. Selye H. The story of the adaptation syndrome. New York: Acta; 1952.
11. Bortz W. The disuse syndrome. West J Med 1984;141:691–9.
12. Peterson P. The gray dawn. New York: Crown Books; 1999.
13. Steel K, Williams TF. Geriatrics: the fruition of the clinician. Arch Intern Med 1974; 134:1125–6.
14. Hayflick L. Aging is no longer an unknown. Ann NY Acad Med 2007;1100:1–13.
15. Zaretsky M. Communication between identical twins, health behavior and social factors are associated with longevity that is greater among identical than fraternal U.S. World War II veteran twins. J Gerontol A Biol Sci Med Sci 2003;58(6):566–72.
16. Martin G. The biology of aging: 1985-2010 and beyond. FASEB J 2011;11: 3756–62.
17. Patel CJ, Rehkopf DH, Leppert JT, et al. Systematic evaluation of environmental and behavioral factors assoc. with all cause mortality in NHANES. Int J Epidemiol 2013;42:1775–810.
18. Bortz W. Redefining human aging. J Am Geriatr Soc 1989;37:1092–6.
19. Wetle T. Age as a risk factor for inadequate treatment. JAMA 1987;256:516.
20. Schrodinger E. What is life? The physical aspects of living cells. New York: Cambridge University Press; 1967.
21. Lunney JR, Lynn J. Trajectory of disability in last year of life. N Engl J Med 2010; 363:294.
22. Medawar P. An unsolved problem of biology lecture. London: University College; 6 December, 1951.
23. Zhang WB, Pincus Z. Predicting all cause mortality from basic physiology in the Framingham Heart Study. Aging Cell 2015;15:39–48.
24. Fried L, Tangen CM, Walston J, et al. The frailty phenotype. J Gerontol A Biol Sci Med Sci 2001;56:M146–56.
25. Bortz W. A conceptual framework of frailty: a review. J Gerontol A Biol Sci Med Sci 2002;57(5):M283–8.
26. Yates FE. Modeling frailty: can a simple feedback model suffice? Mech Ageing Dev 2008;129:671–2.
27. Hoffman P. Life's ratchet. New York: Basic Books; 2012.
28. Prigogine I, Stengers I. Order out of chaos. New York: Bantam; 1984.
29. Weibel E. Symmorphosis: on form and function in shaping life. Cambridge (MA): Harvard University Press; 2000.
30. Bortz W. Aging as entropy. Exp Gerontol 1986;21:321–8.
31. Blair SN, Kohl HW, Paffenbarger RS Jr, et al. Physical fitness and all cause mortality. JAMA 1995;273:1094–100.
32. Fiatarone MA, Marks EC, Ryan ND, et al. Strength training in nonagenarians. JAMA 1990;63:3029–34.

An Elder Care Imperative

Check for updates

Steven D. Johnson, PA-C[a,b,c,*]

KEYWORDS

- Silver tsunami • Physician assistant • Geriatric skill set • Primary care impact

KEY POINTS

- The population of the United States and the world is experiencing an unprecedented geriatric demographic shift, often referred to as the silver tsunami.
- Reasonable predictions suggest a deficit of physicians and, especially, geriatric trained physicians.
- Primary care will assume the main responsibility of managing increasing numbers of time-intensive geriatric patients.
- With a deficit in the physician work force, the physician assistant and the advanced nurse practitioner may be tasked with increasing responsibility for frail medically complex geriatric patients.
- It is reasonable to expect significant challenges to clinic schedules and place of practice with the silver tsunami.
- Primary care providers will need to develop a geriatric skill set that includes cognitive evaluation, functional assessment, pain management, polypharmacy, and end-of-life counseling.

INTRODUCTION

It's tough to make predictions, especially about the future.

—Yogi Berra

I approach this introduction and any prediction regarding the expected population shift of older adults with caution. As an older adult, I can look back on multiple serious predictions that have not had the expected impact on society or medicine.

In college, we read Paul Ehrlich's *The Population Bomb*, which predicted mass starvation by the 1970s and 1980s, and which, thankfully, did not occur.[1]

Disclosure Statement: None.
[a] Stanford University/Foothill Community College, Stanford, CA, USA; [b] Sutter Health, Palo Alto Medical Foundation, Palo Alto Division, The Guzik Family Center for Geriatrics and Palliative Care, 795 El Camino Real, Palo Alto, CA 94301, USA; [c] American Academy of Physician Assistants, Society of Physician Assistants Caring for the Elderly, President, 2318 Mill Road, Ste 1300, Alexandria, VA 22314, USA
* 463 Loma Vista Terrace, Pacifica, CA 94044.
E-mail address: sdeckerjohnson@mac.com

Physician Assist Clin 3 (2018) 469–477
https://doi.org/10.1016/j.cpha.2018.05.001
2405-7991/18/© 2018 Elsevier Inc. All rights reserved.

When I graduated from my grueling physician assistant (PA) training in 1982, the Graduate Medical Education National Advisory Committee report[2] on US physician manpower (sic) policies reported an expected excess of 70,000 physicians by the 1990s and recommended medical schools decrease their enrollment by 10%. For the still new PA graduates, this seemed to predict a certain demise of the profession and few, if any, employment opportunities.

During my training a new, deadly, and untreatable disease was recognized. In 1983, it was identified as the human T-cell lymphotropic virus-type III or lymphadenopathy-associated virus, and later renamed the human immunodeficiency virus (HIV). The prediction for this illness was for rapid population spread. Health care, especially primary care, would be tasked with treating ever-increasing numbers of patients with HIV. No one imagined that within 20 years HIV would be a manageable illness not unlike diabetes.

So, as I consider the expected impact of an aging population on health care, especially primary care, I do so with caution. It is safe to say that there is a population shift to an overall older population. It is not unreasonable to expect that the forefront of medicine, the primary care office, will assume the brunt of the aging demographic. Each day will bring an increasing percentage of older adults with chronic disease and frailty who will require multifaceted management. The primary care providers, including medical doctors, PAs, and advanced practice registered nurses (APRNs), will need to develop a geriatric medicine perspective and skill set to meet the unique needs of older, medically complex, frail adults. For the front-line clinician, managing the time needed to competently address the needs of the frail ill older adult will be critical to success. Time requirements will include time preparing for the visit, time for the scheduled visit, time for the after-visit follow-up, time to coordinate with and listen to family and caregivers, time to address referrals, and time to coordinate social and community services and subspecialists.

AN AGING POPULATION

The prediction and evidence for a demographic shift to an older patient population is compelling. For the first time in world history, the population will shift to more older and retired adults than young, working adults. As the post–World War II baby boom demographic ages, the population of adults older than 65 years is projected to nearly double from 43.1 million in 2012 to more than 83.7 million by 2050.[3] The percentage of adults older than 65 years in 2014 was about 15% and is expected to reach 20% in 2030.[3] In the coming decade, 2020 to 2030, the number of adults older than 65 years is projected to increase by 18,000,000, from approximately 46,000,000 to 64,000,000, which will affect most health care providers in practice today.[4]

Because of the aging population, the location of clinical practice may need to shift from the office into the community. The aging baby boom generation will increase the need for skilled nursing facilities and long-term care by more than 75% from 1.3 million in 2010 to possibly 2.3 million in 2030.[4] In light of the need to reduce hospital readmission rates, the necessity for hands-on evaluations of ill patients in skilled nursing facilities will require nursing home visits. There will be a need for home and community clinic visits, which will shift the locus of office-based practice and bring new challenges.

In light of the aging population, it is necessary to define the term old. Geriatric medicine defines ages greater than 65 years as young-old (65–74 years), middle-old (75–84 years), and old-old or oldest old (85 years and beyond). However, age, the number of years lived, is not necessarily a determinant of health or function. It is important to assess the person in the context of her or his current function and social support. The retired physician at 83 years who still writes, publishes articles and books, runs 3 miles daily, and lectures is a different functional person than the 74-year-old who is immobilized with depression, chronic obstructive pulmonary disease (COPD), and cardiovascular disease. Age is a factor but not the sole determinant of function and health. Although frailty catches up to us all, habits, activity, engagement, and community better define the actual health and function of the person who trusts us with their care.

An expected challenge of the aging population will be an increasing percentage of primarily age-specific diseases into our primary care practices. Alzheimer dementia affects 1 in 10 adults older than 65 years, about 10%. The percentage increases with age, with 3% of people who are young-old (65–74), 17% of people middle-old, and 32% of old-old adults affected by Alzheimer dementia.[5] The time to assess and manage older frail patients with cognitive impairment, and to address family or caregiver questions and concerns, will be significant and, in fact, a schedule buster. Primary care practices may be expected to start to manage ever-increasing numbers of older patients with dementia, which will significantly affect the day-to-day schedule. Think of a primary care schedule with 5 dementia or cognitively impaired patients and family visits every day.

A January 2018 article in *JAMA Neurology* predicts a Parkinson disease (PD) pandemic, "Conservatively applying worldwide prevalence data from a 2014 meta-analysis[6] to projections of the world's future population[7] the number of people with PD will double from 6.9 million in 2015 to 14.2 million in 2040."[8] PD is among the most prevalent neurodegenerative diseases with an age-associated onset. It is reasonable to expect increasing numbers of PD patients in primary care across the country. Often, the coordination of care and community resources, as well as addressing day-to-day clinical problems, will fall to the primary care team. Again, the time demands for management and coordination of care will significantly affect the primary care schedule both during and after clinic hours.

Orthopedic concerns, including common osteoarthritis, joint replacement, and hip fractures, will require thoughtful management to prevent disability, manage pain, address postsurgical rehabilitation, and (often) subsequent disability. Think of a busy clinic day with 18 to 25 patient visits: 6 or 8 patients who are 80-plus years old with renal disease or hypertension, taking 5 or more medications, and/or complaining of joint pain and disability. It is not unreasonable to predict that the day-to-day impact on clinical schedules will be profound.

Last year, the Association of American Medical Colleges (AAMC) published *The Complexities of Physician Supply and Demand 2017 Update: Projections from 2015 to 2030*, complied by IHS Markit. This is the third set of workforce projections by the AAMC to best inform and update policy makers and the health care industry regarding the capacity of the US medical workforce, physicians in particular. The AAMC considers potential scenarios that affect the physician workforce, including physician retirement, changing demographics, and greater integration of APRNs and PAs. The AAMC projects a total physician workforce shortage of between 40,800 and 104,100 physicians by 2030. The AAMC also projects shortfalls in primary care of between 7300 and 43,100 physicians, and in nonprimary care specialties of between 33,500 and 61,800 physicians by 2030.

In a separate publication, the AAMC identified 4833 active geriatric physicians in 2013.[9] There are not sufficient numbers of trained geriatric medicine physicians to manage the current population of older adults. Reasonable projections do not show a dramatic increase of geriatric medicine physicians trained for the expected increase in the older adult population. It is reasonable to expect that the primary responsibility for older adult care will fall to primary care teams.

With a shortfall in the physician workforce, nonphysician providers, PAs and APRNs, will assume those clinical responsibilities by necessity. The influx of older adults, particularly frail older adults, will shift clinical expectations and demands on primary care schedules. Primary care will be tasked with the additional clinical, social, and end-of-life challenges that are expected of a geriatric provider. Primary care teams will need to adjust and continue the critical task of care coordination and interdisciplinary management that is essential not only to better health and lower resource utilization but also to competent health care.

GERIATRIC SKILL SET

In practical terms, care of the frail older population will require the geriatric skill set of cognitive evaluation, management of dementia, screening for depression, functional assessment, managing polypharmacy, managing chronic pain, and addressing end-of-life goals and planning. Often, the focus of elder care is the management of chronic illness while evaluating and maximizing function. It requires a team for each patient that includes specialists, social services, education resources, spouse or partner, family, friends, and community.

The impact of just a few more complex frail adults every day on our practice schedule will be significant. Every patient requires time and careful consideration. We have a professional, moral, and legal mandate to competently interview and assess every person who trusts us with their care. For the medically complex older adult, the time to assess and manage increases exponentially. In the care of older adults, there are multiple clinical considerations that deserve to be addressed and will increasingly fall to the primary care team.

The strength of primary care is the routine visit that builds a relationship with the patient and his or her family, friends, and community. This month-after-month and year-after-year relationship allows for the astute observation of the adult over time. The broad skill base of the primary care provider is ideal for the management of the older and frail older adult. The geriatric challenge to primary care is in shifting the perspective to functional assessment and support, management of polypharmacy, establishing goals for care, functional assessment, cognitive evaluation, and understanding the patient's care community.

Cognitive Evaluation

I am often surprised at patients who have well-established deficits of memory and cognition who enjoy reading and are aware and opinionated about politics and current events. Timing and context are important. Clearly demented patients may participate and engage when family is present and they are clean and comfortable. However, stress, illness, or discomfort exacerbates symptoms of dementia and patients can be incommunicative and withdrawn.

Subtle changes in cognition and behavior require thoughtful evaluation. A broad differential diagnosis that always includes infection and medication misadventure is critical to catching early presenting illness, perhaps before a trip to the emergency room is needed. Primary care relationships that develop over time are critical to prevention of cascading clinical catastrophes, such as a urinary tract infection or upper respiratory infection, leading to dehydration and exacerbation of mild cognitive decline, ranging from confusion to wandering to fall and fracture. The well-understood cascade of events will demand clinician availability, team work, coordination, and time as the number of frail elders increases in each primary care practice.

The Montreal Cognitive Assessment (MoCA) and the Mini-Mental Status Examination (MMSE) are useful in evaluating and documenting cognitive function in the primary care setting. The tests can be administered by support staff and evaluated by the clinician.

Depression

I recently cared for a 99-year-old frail but cognitively intact woman who firmly explained to me that aging, especially the extremes of age, is characterized by loss. She lost her husband, all of her friends, and 2 of her children. Illness, loss of family and friends, declining function, and caregiver strain, can often lead to depression. Careful attention to mood, activity changes, nonspecific complaints, and fatigue can lead to clinical exploration of depression. Routine screening with a validated depression scale, such as the Patient Health Questionnaire (PHQ)-3 or PHQ-9, is an important part of addressing depression in the older adult population.

Medication Review and Polypharmacy

Comprehensive medication management is essential to successful care of the older adult. Adverse drug reactions (ADRs) account for significant morbidity and hospitalizations in the older adult population. There are 2 kinds of ADR, which are defined by Rawlings and Thompson[10] as type A and type B. Type A reaction is dose-dependent and predictable. For instance, warfarin adjusted without monitoring; antibiotics given without recent renal function assessment; hypoglycemia from insulin; drug-related orthostatic hypotension, resulting in falls and fractures; gastrointestinal bleeding from nonsteroidal antiinflammatory drug medications, prescribed and over-the-counter; and delirium from pain, psychiatric, and insomnia medications are a few examples. Type B is the idiosyncratic reaction that is not predictable, such as a florid allergic reaction to a previously tolerated medication or Steven-Johnson syndrome. Type A reactions are the most common by far. Of hospitalized older adults, 10% have an identified ADR versus 6.3% of younger patients.[11] It was recently reported that 60% of nursing home residents experience an ADR.[12,13] Almost every clinician I know has the experience of reviewing an older adult's medication list and the gut-wrenching surprise of finding high-risk medications, unmonitored medications, or potential medication interactions that have not been recognized during the routine course of treatment by multiple providers.

Every visit should include a review of prescribed medications and supplements. It is important to understand alternative therapies that an older adult has chosen to pursue or are being given by well-meaning friends and family members. It is not uncommon to discover that patients will share medications with friends. The specifics of what a person is actually taking (vs what is prescribed) are critical to the prevention of unintended complications and side effects. Many providers insist that older adults bring in all their medications and supplements in a brown bag so the clinical staff can not only record which medications are being taken but also if they are taken, how many are left, and if the family and patient understand why the medications are prescribed and how to effectively take them. Of course, reviewing a bag of 6 medications and 5 supplements, discussing side effects and dangers, then reconciling the medications in the electronic medical record during a 15-minute scheduled visit is a challenge for any provider. It is important to engage the care team across specialties to understand the goals of clinical care and potential medication side effects and interactions. If possible, family members need to be included in the conversation; they often have insight to actual medication use versus prescribed medication schedule.

Although all medication and supplements have potential side effects, every provider caring for older adults, especially the complex elderly, should have a mental stop sign when patients have been prescribed anticoagulants, antihypertensive, diuretics, and/or insulin. These are the most common medications to cause unintended complications, medication interactions, and adverse outcomes.

The American Geriatric Society publishes a list of high-risk medications for the elderly, "Beers Criteria for Potentially Inappropriate Medication Use in Older Adults." Named after the late geriatric physician Mark Beers, MD, this is an invaluable reference table for primary care providers to review and assess potentially preventable medication side effects for older adults.

It is critical to assess the hepatic and renal clearance for older adults and adjust medications accordingly. Keep in mind the fluctuation of renal function with acute illness and dehydration.

Function is Primary

For younger patients, the medical visit is to address a specific illness or injury, or for preventive screening. For the older adult, management of chronic illness in the context of independent function and quality of life is more often the focus. The challenge for the clinician is to manage chronic and acute medical illness within the context of maximizing function. The advantage of the primary care relationship is the ability to assess function over time, which allows a critical perspective on gradual or abrupt decline of ability or mentation.

Assessing activities of daily living (ADL) and instrumental ADL (IADL) is the basis for assessing function in the older adult. ADL include toileting, feeding, dressing, grooming, physical ambulation, and bathing. IADL include the ability to use telephone, shop, prepare food, do housekeeping, do laundry, manage transportation, be responsible for one's medication, and to manage finances.

However, function for older adults is multifaceted. Emotional state is important and depression is common for adults who have faced significant loss over a lifetime. Cognitive function is critical to maintaining independence and requires thoughtful observation during every clinical encounter. Community activities are a measure of function. Knowledge of a patient's ability to attend and participate at church, movies, concerts, theater, or other community activities is important for the clinician to best understand function. These are often the activities that give meaning to daily life and are critical to support when interventions are considered. A sudden change in usual community activities is a red flag for the clinician, as is a change in function and health.

Function is more important than age. In considering recovery from influenza or pneumonia, the professor who walks his dog 3 miles every day, plays bridge, and continues to teach at 88 years of age is a clinically different patient than the 72-year-old who has endstage renal disease, COPD, and poorly controlled diabetes. Understanding function allows for thoughtful consideration of what can be expected after an unexpected injury or illness, and allows the clinician to counsel the patient and family on reasonable expectations for recovery.

Pain Management

We are in the midst of a national tragedy with an opioid addiction crisis. Addiction does not spare the elderly. However, aging often entails pain. Managing pain requires careful and judicious use of multiple agents and modalities to alleviate chronic discomfort and enhance function. A recent patient of mine suffered from endstage disabling hip pain from bone-on-bone osteoarthritis. She was unable to walk, suffered agony to stand and transfer to wheelchair or toilet, and was unable to sleep with nighttime pain. She had avoided opioid medications for years owing to an allergy. With a careful family history and chart review, we found that in years past she had tolerated hydromorphone (Dilaudid) on several occasions without significant cognitive or allergic side effects. After a careful, lengthy review of risks and potential benefits with the patient and her family, I prescribed a routine dose of hydromorphone. Within 2 days, she was sleeping well, was more mobile, and was dramatically more comfortable and happy. Now, when I pass her in the hallway, she greets me with a smile, often a ribald joke, and a detailed report of her sleep and mobility. Although she is improved, she will not heal. This is the nature of geriatric care; she will require close follow-up, monitoring, and adjustment of medication regime. As she continues her aging journey, the potential for serious complications, including constipation, falls, and confusion, also increases and can only be monitored through careful partnership with her and her family and caregivers.

Care Community

Because most adults age in place, their independent function often relies on a community of caregivers. Care of the elderly requires an understanding of this informal and sometimes formal social support system. Who does the cooking, who goes to the store, who cleans the home, and who does the laundry? Who drives? If the older adult drives, are they safe to drive? Understanding community support services, such as Meals on Wheels, local senior centers, and adult daycare services, is important to assessing function and supporting function for isolated older adults. Spouse, family, friends, neighbors, and paid caregivers should be included, when appropriate, in care plans.

To understand the network of support that an older adults rely on allows insight into their cognitive function and their ability to make their needs known. Including the caregivers allows for a better understanding of the limits of an older adult's function. In my skilled nursing facility practice, clinical insight repeatedly comes from simply sharing with the nursing assistants who provide day-to-day personal care. The care community is a complex social structure around each of us, especially older adults. They may be as simple as a dedicated spouse or as complex as community resources and caring neighbors providing resources to keep an adult in their home.

Goals of Care

A critical aspect of elder care is to clarify and define what extent of care should be provided. The conversation about the goals of care is actually an ongoing discussion about wishes; desires; and, often, the stark reality of aging, illness, and death.

It is important to begin the conversation with open-ended questions to allow patients to consider and best express their concerns and understanding of what they want in the context of their current health. Sometimes it is vague and undefined; for instance, they may want to live as long as possible. Sometimes it is specific; they may want live for 1 more Christmas, family birthday, graduation, or birth of a grandchild. Each is a starting point that allows the clinician to reflect, educate, and problem-solve. Providers often focus on the details of cardiopulmonary resuscitation, intubation, and intensive care unit care, and if each is desired or appropriate. In my experience, each adult wants appropriate intervention if there is a reasonable chance of recovery of function and joy. If the outcome will be only pain and discomfort, or a greatly diminished consciousness, most adults only wish for pain management and comfort care. It is important to define the specifics, to complete the Physician Orders for Life Sustaining Treatment (POLST) forms and advance directives, and to reassure both patient and family that whatever the goals, care continues, even if that care is focused on comfort medications and supportive care while the patient is dying.

It is common to have dissenters, such as family members who adamantly oppose the expressed desires of the patient. Reviewing the functional capacity of the patient and the patient's expressed wishes may allow a process of understanding and possibly reconciliation with the reality of the clinical situation.

Patient Autonomy

Fundamentally, every person expresses the need for autonomy and independence. The older adult, in particular, faces small losses each year: the loss of strength, including difficulty opening jars, decreased stamina, the danger of falling, and the advent of illness; the loss of mobility, including the loss of the independence of driving; and, for some, dementia or the loss of self. For the clinician, it is always difficult to be between a family who sees decline and a patient who only sees loss.

Part of autonomy is the legal right to make poor health care choices. The patient may choose to return home where the support is tenuous at best; to ignore dietary requirements or avoid taking prescribed medications; to refuse needed clinical evaluations, follow-up visits, or care plans; or to continue to smoke. Often these stubborn, sometimes fearful, patient refusals result in exacerbations of illness and repeated returns to the emergency room. Supporting our patients may require restraint on our part when they make decisions that are not in their best interest. When confronted with stubborn intent, it is important to engage the support community, to develop contingency plans, to counsel and advise, and then to let go and be ready to again engage when they decline. The age-old strategy is to retreat and retry, again and again, and offer care and guidance when we can.

Time

I do not believe any of the elder care considerations previously discussed are unknown or unexpected by any experienced clinician. The critical issue for the expected shift to an older population is the requirement of time: time to evaluate, time to discuss, time to interview the patient and their family and caregivers, time to listen to worries and fears, and time to review each medication. Then, more time is required, to question, *Should I have done this, checked a laboratory result, or stopped that medication?* Time is required to examine and chart.

Time is required to counsel, to understand a person's wishes, to work with concerned family and friends, and to set up contingency plans. If your clinical life has been anything like mine, with the ever-increasing demands for productivity, decreasing reimbursement, increasing electronic medical record requirements (and, importantly, upgrades), and shifting staff expectations, then the clinical expectations of adding 2 or 5 or 8 more frail adults to daily practice is simply unimaginable and even alarming.

The expectation of a single provider doing it all is coming to a close. The complexity of patient care, the astonishing pace of medical science and clinical algorithms, combined with rapid technological advances and demands of the electronic medical record in a fractured health care system is overwhelming. Teams of clinicians, working in concert, using the extent of their individual training and skills, will be critical to address the coming shift of clinical demands and elder care expectations.

SUMMARY

Predictions are fraught with uncertainty. However, the data for a significantly older patient population combined with expected shortages of physicians are compelling. These changes will affect clinical practices in the next 10, 15, and 20 years. The demands of 96 million baby boomer adults will be experienced by all of us: those in practice and those who are retiring into a health care system stressed by this expected population shift. Now is the time to give consideration to this expected shift. Now is the time for social and political action. Now is the time to plan for the challenges of the silver tsunami. Now is the geriatric imperative.

REFERENCES

1. Ehrlich PR. The Population Bomb. Sierra Club/Ballantine Books, 1968.
2. Report of the Graduate Medical Education National Advisory Committee to the Secretary, Department of Health and Human Services. Volume 1; Health Resources Administration (DHHS/PHS), Office of Graduate Medical Education. Hyattsville, MD.
3. Ortman JM, Velkoff, Victoria A. Hogan, Howard in an aging nation: the older population in the United States; current population reports. U.S. Department of Commerce, Economics and Statistics Administration. Suitland (MD): U.S. Census Bureau; 2014. p. 1.
4. Mather M, Jacobson LA, Pollard KM. Population reference bureau. Popul Bull 2015;70(2):3, 5.
5. Alzheimer's Association. Alzheimer's disease facts and figures. p. 20. 2017.
6. Pringsheim T, Jette N, Frolkis A, et al. The prevalence of Parkinson's disease: a systematic review and meta-analysis. Mov Disord 2014;29(13):1583–90.
7. US Census Bureau. International programs: region summary. Available at: www.cnesus.gov/population/international/data/idb/region/php. Accessed September 29, 2017.
8. Dorsey ER, Bloem BR. The Parkinson pandemic-A call to action. JAMA Neurol 2018;75(1):9–10.
9. Association of American Medical Colleges. 2014 physician specialty data book, center for workforce studies. Washington, (DC): Association of American Medical Colleges; 2014. p. 8.
10. Rawlings MD, Thompson JP. Pathogenesis of adverse drug reactions. In: Davis DM, editor. Textbook of adverse drug reactions. Oxford (United Kingdom): Oxford University Press; 1977. p. 44.
11. Konkaew C, Noyce PL, Ashcroft D. Hospital admissions associated with adverse drug reactions: a systematic review of prospective observational studies. Ann Pharmacother 2008;42:1017–25.
12. Dilles T, Vander Stichele R, Van Bortel L, et al. The development and test of an intervention to improve ADR screening in nursing homes. J Am Med Dir Assoc 2013;14:317–76.
13. American Geriatrics Society 2015 Updated Beers Criteria for Potentially Inappropriate Medication Use in Older Adults. Journal of the American Geriatric Society 2015;63(11):2227–46.

Evaluation and Management of Falls

Kathy Kemle, MS, PA-C[a,b,*], Dipesh Patel, MD[a]

KEYWORDS

- Falls • Geriatric syndromes • Interventions for falls • Evaluation of fallers

KEY POINTS

- Falls are a growing public health crisis in the United States that requires the commitment of every health care provider to reduce their occurrence and impact on individuals and the society.
- Risk factors for falls are readily identifiable during health care encounters and should be routinely assessed, especially in cognitively impaired individuals.
- As a geriatric syndrome, falls are multifactorial and require an interdisciplinary team for optimal management.
- Maintenance of visual acuity and group exercise programs that include balance, strength training, and resistance training hold the best hope for reducing injuries from falls.

INTRODUCTION AND EPIDEMIOLOGY

Unintentional falls are the leading cause of fatal and nonfatal injuries among adults 65 years of age and older. In 2016, falls resulted in more than 29,000 deaths, and nonfatal falls resulted in approximately 285,000 subsequent hospitalizations, costing more than $9 billion. Unfortunately, as the population continues to age, the number of annual adult falls and their costs are projected to increase, reaching more than $100 billion by 2030.[1] This amount does not include the psychological and other costs to patients and caregivers, because falls often precipitate dramatic declines in function, leading to a need for increasing levels of care and, often, nursing home placement.

As primary care providers, physician assistants are in the vanguard of efforts to reduce this growing public health dilemma. A working knowledge of the factors and diagnoses associated with falls, together with a targeted history and physical examination, can identify those most at risk. Interventions aimed at the individual's unique

Disclosure Statement: Nothing to disclose.
[a] Division of Geriatrics, Department of Family Medicine, Medical Center of Central Georgia, Navicent Health, 3780 Eisenhower Parkway, Macon, GA 31206, USA; [b] Family Health Center, 3780 Eisenhower Parkway, Macon, GA 31206, USA
* Corresponding author. Family Health Center, 3780 Eisenhower Parkway, Macon, GA 31206.
E-mail address: tivolikw@aol.com

Physician Assist Clin 3 (2018) 479–486
https://doi.org/10.1016/j.cpha.2018.05.002
2405-7991/18/© 2018 Elsevier Inc. All rights reserved.

fall profile can mitigate the risk for many persons. Referral to other members of the interdisciplinary team and community resources completes the multipronged approach needed for effective reduction in fall injuries.

Risk Factors Associated with Falling

Falls are a geriatric syndrome and thus are multifactorial in origin. They result from combinations of intrinsic factors inherent within the individual and extrinsic ones within the environment. For example, an older woman with lower-extremity osteoarthritis, visual impairment, and urinary incontinence who rushes through a cluttered bedroom to the slippery floor of a bathroom with throw rugs is almost guaranteed to fall at some point. Clinicians must be alert to the complex interaction between individuals and their surroundings.

Numerous studies have focused on risks associated with falls, but most are limited in scope or include only certain populations, such as long-term care patients. In 2017, the first study to look at a large population of older community dwellers evaluated insurance claims over a 1-year period to predict falls within the subsequent 2 years. Echoing other reports, they found that female gender and increasing age, especially those older than 85 years, predicted falls. Cognitive disorders and schizophrenia were found to be strongly associated with greater risk. Degenerative neurologic conditions, central nervous system (CNS) infections, seizure disorders, mood disorders, and syncope as well as sleep disorders and anxiety conferred more than 2 times the risk. Certain medications, especially antidementia agents, dopaminergic agents, antipsychotics, antidepressants, diuretics, and surprisingly, laxatives, increased risk. Polypharmacy also increased the risk by producing drug interactions that increase adverse effects. Drug metabolism changes as part of normal aging with some decline in hepatic and renal elimination of many agents. An increase in fat-to-lean ratio also changes drug distribution, which may result in toxicity.[2] However, Homer and colleagues[3] found that demographics and diagnoses accounted for the greatest degree of elevated risk. **Box 1** lists the Intrinsic and Extrinsic Factors associated with falls.

Complications

Fallers face numerous complications and injuries. They may suffer lacerations, fractures, and traumatic brain injury as well as death. Hip fractures are associated with more than twice the usual death rate within 1 year, and mortality remains elevated for more than 8 years thereafter.[4] Some deaths are directly related to the fall, but many are the final common pathway of increasing frailty related to age, disease, and disuse.

Other less obvious complications include a decline in independence and ability to complete instrumental and basic activities of daily living. Such functional declines may result in long-term care placement for those without adequate social support. Some patients develop a deep fear of falling (fallophobia) and may limit their activity attempting to limit their risk. Ironically, this usually increases their susceptibility because immobility causes sarcopenia, as well as poorer standing and dynamic balance, contributing to more serious fall injuries.

EVALUATION OF THE OLDER ADULT WHO HAS FALLEN
History

As in many clinical syndromes, the key to arriving at the causes of a fall is a thorough history. If the person presents with a fall, inquire about their last fall and prior falls. It is

> **Box 1**
> **Risk factors for falls**
>
> *Intrinsic*
>
> - Age/female gender
> - Diagnoses
> - Medications
> - Frailty
> - Fallophobia
> - Visual impairment
> - History of prior fall
>
> *Extrinsic*
>
> - Environmental factors
> - Poor lighting
> - Slippery surfaces
> - Clutter, obstacles
> - Inappropriate footwear
> - Improper use of or inappropriate assistive devices
> - Polypharmacy or psychoactive drugs

best to phrase the question presupposing that the older adult has fallen and ask in an open-ended manner. For example, "Tell me about the last time you fell, even if you did not injure yourself," removes the embarrassment associated with falling and signals your desire to help the older adult avoid falling in the future. A similar question is helpful for persons whom you are screening in an effort to reduce future falls, because most people who suffer injuries had at least one noninjurious fall before that event.

Solicit any prodromal symptoms, such as dizziness or vertigo. Ask for a description of the circumstances of the fall, injuries, and contributing environmental factors. Assess for possibly vagal stimulation as a cause; for example, straining at stool or urinating against obstruction. Beware of those who report a slip or trip as the only cause. Some older adults may not remember the event and will assume they suffered an environmental mishap. Review risk factors with the patient, their diagnoses, medications, including over the counter and supplements, and investigate visual acuity, cognition, gait, and balance. Does the patient report feeling unsteady when arising or walking? Do they use an assistive device such as a walker or cane? **Boxes 2–4** list diseases and medications commonly associated with fall risk. Remember that all of the factors are at least additive and possibly synergistic.

Physical Examination

Evaluate for orthostatic hypotension by measuring blood pressure (BP) and pulse in multiple positions. Measure the supine BP and pulse, after the patient has been lying down for 5 minutes. Next, repeat the readings after the individual has been sitting for one to 2 minutes. Last, repeat them after the patient has been standing for one to 2 minutes. Orthostatic hypotension is noted with a decrease in systolic BP greater than 20 mm Hg and/or a decline in diastolic of 10 mm Hg. Hypovolemia may be signaled

Box 2
Diagnoses associated with falls

- Hepatic/renal disease
- Autonomic dysfunction
- Cognitive impairment
- Stroke
- Depression
- Seizure disorder
- Anxiety/mood disorders
- Diabetes mellitus with neuropathy/other peripheral neuropathies
- Malaise
- Alcohol use
- Vitamin D deficiency
- Parkinson and its variants
- Postural hypotension
- Urinary incontinence
- Severe lower extremity osteoarthritis
- Schizophrenia
- Degenerative neurologic disorders
- Visual disorders
- Conduction disorders
- CNS infections
- Delirium
- Acute illness

by an increase in the pulse of greater than 30 beats per minute. Lightheadedness or dizziness on standing also suggests orthostatic hypotension.[5] It should be noted that orthostatic hypotension has been found to be associated with first but not subsequent falls.[6]

Evaluate visual acuity and peripheral vision. A mild decline in peripheral vision is normal, but visual field cuts require further evaluation by an ophthalmologist, as

Box 3
General medications associated with fall risk

- Sedatives/hypnotics
- Antidepressants
- Neuroleptics
- Acetylcholinesterase inhibitors
- Diabetic agents (hypoglycemia)
- Anticonvulsants

Box 4
Anticholinergic medications associated with falls

- Antihistamines, especially first generation, like diphenhydramine
- Oxybutynin and other overactive bladder agents
- Tricyclic antidepressants
- Promethazine
- Anti-Parkinsonian
- Nonsteroidal anti-inflammatories
- Calcium channel blockers
- Loop diuretics
- Alpha-blockers
- Digoxin

---

does the presence of cataracts. A thorough cardiac examination including a search for murmurs and carotid bruits should be done. However, most bruits are NOT associated with cerebral insufficiency and heightened fall risk. Evaluate gait and balance, both standing and dynamic, as well as proprioception and deep tendon reflexes. Lower-extremity strength and range of motion should be examined. A simple and easily performed gait evaluation is the Tinetti Up and Go Test, which requires the person to rise from a chair, preferably without using their arms, walk 10 feet, turn, and return to the chair and sit down (see section on screening for more detail on the Tinetti test).

An indispensable part of the examination is the cognitive status of the individual. Psychiatric illnesses and cognitive impairment are strongly associated with falls. For a quick evaluation, the Mini-Cog, which includes a 3-item recall and clock drawing test, is helpful, but is only a screen and not necessarily diagnostic of dementia. Delirium is also associated with falls, but may be missed, especially if the person is exhibiting the hypoactive form. It is characterized by inattention, variability in severity of symptoms, disordered thinking, and a change in level of consciousness. There are several screening instruments, but the most commonly used is the Confusion Assessment Method introduced by Dr Sharon Inouye and colleagues.[7] Delirium should be aggressively considered and managed. As a geriatric syndrome, it is multifactorial and associated with medications (many the same as those associated with falls), medical disorders, sensory impairment, electrolyte imbalances, hypoglycemia, and, hypoxemia, to name but a few of the most common causes.

Laboratory and Diagnostic Evaluation

Basic laboratories should include thyroid stimulating hormone and vitamin B12 (cyanocobalamin) because both are associated with peripheral neuropathy. A complete blood count, looking for anemia or possibly an occult infection, is usually done. A comprehensive metabolic panel, including electrolytes, plus renal and hepatic function is appropriate. Serum 25-hydroxy-vitamin D should be performed because deficiency is associated with muscle weakness and falling. Based on history and physical findings, consider electrocardiogram, Holter monitoring, or ambulatory BP monitoring. If cerebral-vascular disease is suspected or if significant head injury has occurred, a computed tomographic brain scan without contrast may be needed.

INTERVENTIONS TO PREVENT FALLS AND THEIR ASSOCIATED INJURIES
General

Reduction of fall risk and related injuries requires a comprehensive approach, screening to target those most at risk, while evaluating and intervening in intrinsic and extrinsic risks.

Screening

The American Geriatrics Society recommends screening for falls annually in all adults 65 years of age or older.[8] Ask individuals about their last fall, prior falls, and instability of gait or balance. There are several screening tools available. The Centers for Disease Control and Prevention (CDC) recommends using the Stay Independent brochure and the Stopping Elderly Accidents, Deaths, and Injuries, with a further more comprehensive assessment if either is positive. The Stay Independent Brochure incorporates 12 questions, which may be completed by the patient, if he or she is able to read or by the clinician or nurse. The brochure, an algorithm for screening, evaluation, and intervention, and a pocket guide for fall prevention for health care providers are available at https://www.cdc.gov/steadi/materials.html (**Fig. S1**).

There are other screening tests in the literature, but there is insufficient evidence to recommend one versus another. One that is easily administered, the Tinetti Up and Go test, is also very quickly done, usually taking less than 1 minute, and may be completed by a nurse or medical assistant. Patients are asked to rise from a chair without using their arms, walk 10 feet, turn, return to the chair, and sit down. If the examiner observes unsteadiness, inability to rise from the chair without relying on the arms, loss of balance on turning, or difficulty reassuming the seated position, this suggests a need for further testing. This test is also used in a timed version, with slower times associated with elevated fall risk and a need for more thorough evaluation. A video from the CDC that demonstrates the Timed Up and Go Test can be accessed at https://www.youtube.com/watch?v=BAZY_oLEIGY.

There are further tests to assess balance. The easiest to use in clinical practice is the Four-Stage Test (FSBT), which requires the patient to demonstrate ability to progress through challenging positions: feet side by side, semitandem stance, one foot directly in front of the other (tandem gait), and standing on one foot. An older adult who cannot maintain tandem stance for more than 10 seconds is at increased risk for falls. A video of the FSBT can be accessed at https://www.youtube.com/watch?v=3HvMLLIGY6c. Individuals who fail these basic screening tests should be referred for further evaluation by a physical therapist.

MEDICATION REVIEW, SUPPLEMENTATION, AND EXERCISE PROGRAMS

Other needed interventions include appropriate medication review and discontinuation of potentially offending drugs. See **Box 2** for those most associated with increased risk. Vitamin D deficiency is common in older adults, and levels should be assessed to guide therapy. Vitamin D supplementation to a serum 25-hydroxy-vitamin D level of at least 30 ng/mL is recommended by the American Geriatrics Society.[9] However, vitamin D and calcium supplementation without documented deficiency has not been shown to reduce hip fractures, vertebral fractures, or other such injuries, when used as a single intervention in community dwelling older adults.[10] Exercise programs that incorporate group training, balance and strength training, and resistance training show the best evidence for efficacy.[11] Yoga and tai chi have been shown to be beneficial in several studies.[11,12] Walking as a single intervention, while certainly better than no exercise, has not been shown to reduce risk.

VISUAL IMPAIRMENT/PODIATRIC ISSUES

Visual impairment should be corrected via cataract extraction and/or use of eye-glasses. Antislip shoes, not slippers, and attention to foot deformities, such as bunions and lengthy toenails, are simple measures that can be surprisingly effective.

EXTRINSIC FACTOR MODIFICATION

Environmental modification to reduce hazards within the home should be recommended, and a visit by an occupational therapist is useful to provide guidance for patients and caregivers. If a therapist is not available, the CDC produces a booklet, Home Safety Checklist, which patients and families may use to identify potential dangers in the home. It is available at https://www.cdc.gov/steadi/pdf/check_for_safety_brochure-a.pdf. Common hazards include loose throw rugs, fraying carpet edges, inadequate lighting, poorly maintained stairs lacking guard rails or with high step risers, and a lack of bathroom grab bars. Modifications are often overlooked, but are effective in reducing the rate of falls, especially for those at greatest risk. Although home emergency response systems do not reduce the risk of falls, they may be beneficial in avoiding prolonged "time on ground."[13] Persons who remain down without assistance for an excessive period of time have higher mortality and morbidity.

Those who use assistive devices, such as wheelchairs, canes, or walkers, are at increased risk for falls. Patients may not recognize an ill-fitting or inappropriate device, which may actually increase their risk of an injury. Physical therapists can evaluate the individual, suggest an appropriate and well-fitted device, and instruct the patient in proper use, reducing fall risk.

Hip protectors are hard shields or padded inserts placed in or on specially designed underwear. They may reduce the risk of hip fracture but not the frequency of falls. In nursing home populations, hip protectors have been found to decrease hip fracture incidence slightly but at a cost of increasing pelvic fractures. They are difficult to clean, fit, and maintain and so have not been widely used.[14,15]

SUMMARY

Falls are a grave danger to the health and independence of older adults. They are multifactorial and must be addressed in a comprehensive manner. Although this is a complex process, tools are available to simplify the evaluation and reduce the time needed to perform it. Physician assistants must embrace their role in preventing falls and their related injuries.

SUPPLEMENTARY DATA

Supplementary data related to this article can be found online at https://doi.org/10.1016/j.cpha.2018.05.002.

REFERENCES

1. Houry D, Baldwin G, Stevens J, et al. The CDC injury center's response to the growing public health problem of falls among older adults. Am J Lifestyle Med 2016;10:74–7.
2. Chen Y, Zhu LL, Zhow Q. Effects of drug pharmacokinetic/pharmacodynamic properties, characteristics of medication use, and relevant pharmacological interventions on fall risk in elderly patients. Ther Clin Risk Manag 2014;10:437–48.

3. Homer ML, Palmer NP, Fox KP, et al. Predicting falls in people aged 65 years and older from insurance claims. Am J Med 2017;130(6):744.e17-23.
4. Katsoulis M, Benetou V, Karapetyan T, et al. Excess mortality after hip fracture in elderly persons from Europe and the USA: the CHANCES project. J Intern Med 2017;281(3):300–10.
5. Spector W, Limcangco R. Tool 3F: orthostatic vital sign measurement. Rockville (MD): Agency for Healthcare Research and Quality; 2013. Available at: http://www.ahrq.gov/professionals/systems/hospital/fallpxtoolkit/fallpxtk-tool3f.html.
6. Hartog LC, Schrijnders D, Landman GWD, et al. Is orthostatic hypotension related to falling? A meta-analysis of individual patient data of prospective observational studies. Age Ageing 2017;46(4):568–75.
7. Inouye SK, vanDyck CH, Alessi CA, et al. Clarifying confusion: the confusion assessment method. A new method for detection of delirium. Ann Intern Med 1990;113:941–8. Confusion Assessment Method: Training Manual and Coding Guide, Copyright © 2003, Hospital Elder Life Program, LLC.
8. American Geriatrics Society/British Geriatrics Society clinical practice guideline: prevention of falls in older persons. New York: American Geriatrics Society; 2010. Available at: https://geriatricscareonline.org/Product Abstract/updated-american-geriatrics-society/british-geriatrics- society-clinical -practice-guideline-for-prevention-of falls-in-older-persons-and-recommendations/CL014.
9. American Geriatrics Society Workgroup on Vitamin D supplementation for Older Adults. Recommendations abstracted from the American Geriatrics Society Consensus Statement on Vitamin D for Prevention of Falls and Their Consequences. J Am Geriatr Soc 2014;62(1):147–52.
10. Zhao JG, Zeng XT, Wang J, et al. Association between calcium or vitamin D supplementation and fracture incidence in community-dwelling older adults: a systematic review and meta-analysis. JAMA 2017;318(24):2466–82.
11. de Labra C, Guimaraes-Pinheiro C, Maseda A, et al. Effects of physical exercise interventions in frail older adults: a systematic review and meta-analysis of randomized controlled trials. BMC Geriatr 2015;15:154.
12. Voukelatos A, Cumming RG, Lord SR, et al. A randomized controlled trial of tai chi for the prevention of falls: the Central Sydney tai chi trial. J Am Geriatr Soc 2007; 55(8):1185–91.
13. Youkhana S, Dean CM, Wolff M. Yoga-based exercise improves balance and mobility in people aged 60 and over: a systematic review and meta-analysis. Age Ageing 2016;45(1):21–9.
14. Santesso N, Carrasco-Labra A, Brignardello-Petersen R. Hip protectors for preventing hip fractures in older people. Cochrane Database Syst Rev 2014;(3):CD001255.
15. Roush RE, Teasdale TA, Murphy JN, et al. Impact of a personal emergency response system on hospital utilization by community-residing elders. South Med J 1995;88(9):917–22.

Cognitive Decline and Dementia
Primary Care Evaluation and When to Refer

Freddi Segal-Gidan, PA, PhD

KEYWORDS

- Cognitive impairment • Dementia • Mental status • Detection • Evaluation

KEY POINTS

- Cognitive impairment in older adults is underrecognized and dementia is underdiagnosed by providers in primary care.
- Early detection of cognitive impairment in older adults can improve care, reduce complications, and potentially reduce costs.
- Validated tools to screen for depression, mental status, and function are readily available, easy to use, and can easily be incorporated into regular care of older adults.
- A basic evaluation for memory or thinking complaints to identify treatable conditions should be part of primary care.

INTRODUCTION

Cognitive decline is not a normal part of aging; however, with increased age, the risk for development of impairment in memory and other areas of cognitive function increases significantly. Dementia is present in 10% of the population older than age 65 years; by age 85 years up to 40% to 50% of the population have some degree of cognitive impairment.[1] Alzheimer disease, the most common form of dementia in later life, is the sixth leading cause of death in persons older than age 65 years in the United States.[2]

Primary care providers are in an ideal position to identify early signs of cognitive decline in their older patients. However, identification of cognitive impairment in primary care settings is challenging owing to competing priorities, time constraints,

Disclosure: No commercial funding support. Partial support through the National Institutes of Health (NIH), the National Institute on Aging (NIA)-funded University of Southern California (USC) Alzheimers Disease Research Center (ADRC), and the Health Resources and Services Administration (HRSA)-funded USC Geriatric Workforce Project (GWEP).
Keck School of Medicine, University of Southern California, Rancho Los Amigos National Rehabilitation Center, Rancho/USC California Alzheimers Disease Center, 7601 East Imperial Highway, Downey, CA 90242, USA
E-mail address: segalgi@usc.edu

Physician Assist Clin 3 (2018) 487–494
https://doi.org/10.1016/j.cpha.2018.05.003
2405-7991/18/© 2018 Elsevier Inc. All rights reserved.

physicianassistant.theclinics.com

and the additional burdens a dementia diagnosis presents to both patients and providers. Stigma concerns among providers, patients, and families around mental illness and dementia are common and add to the challenge of early detection. Increased awareness among providers can improve early identification and the opportunity to prevent problems that may arise when there is a failure to recognize, diagnose, and develop an appropriate care plan.

Early identification of cognitive impairment can have multiple benefits. When patients with mild cognitive impairment (MCI) or early dementia are identified there is the opportunity for the person with the condition to be actively involved in their future care planning. Benefits of early detection are:

- If negative, alleviation of concerns, reassurance, and decreased anxiety
- If positive, further evaluation, which can result in
  - Identification and treatment of underlying disease or condition
  - Improved management of comorbidities
  - Identification of safety issues (eg, medication management, driving, emergency preparedness)
  - Involvement of patient in long-term care planning (eg, identification of caregiver, creation or update of advance directives, financial and legal planning)
  - Participation in clinical research.

Even though there are currently no disease-modifying treatments, initiation of medications currently approved by the US Food and Drug Administration (FDA) earlier in the course of a neurodegenerative decline offers greater potential to improve symptoms and delay disease progression. The usual practice is to begin with a acetylcholinesterase inhibitor (ie, donepezil, rivastigmine, or galantamine) and then to add memantine to the regimen after a year or 2, depending on the patient's response and disease course. Although these medications are approved for use in Alzheimer disease, they are also often used in other dementias (ie, Lewy Body, vascular, or multi-infarct) but not for frontotemporal lobar dementia.

SCREENING

Impaired cognition among older patients in primary care is underrecognized.[3] Studies have shown that physicians failed to recognize 40% of their cognitively impaired patients and half of patients with dementia had not received a clinical cognitive evaluation.[4,5]

Routine screening for cognitive impairment is currently not recommended. With the growing older population, screening of those older than age 80 years has been suggested as worthwhile.[6] The Medicare wellness visit includes a requirement for the detection of cognitive impairment, which provides an opportunity for screening and early detection. However, there is no specification on how this should be conducted nor is a specific tool recommended.[7]

Few patients mention issues of memory concerns about themselves. Usually it is a family member (eg, spouse, child) who brings their concern to the attention of a medical provider. Office staff can be useful in proactively identifying patients with possible cognitive impairment. Receptionists frequently know which patients forget appointments, even with reminders; show up for an appointment on a wrong day or when none is scheduled; or call repeatedly asking the same question. Medical assistants may be aware of patients who repeat information, fail to make or keep appointments for testing or referrals, or who frequently misplace medications and require additional refills.

When raised by a patient or family member, concerns about changes in memory or thinking should be taken seriously. A brief series of 3 questions (**Box 1**) have been validated and shown useful in detecting cognitive impairment in a general population.[8] A positive answer to any of these questions indicates a need for further evaluation and assessment. The Ascertain Dementia 8-item Informant Questionnaire (AD8), a brief written questionnaire that can be completed by an informant, has been shown to be a reliable screening tool.[9] The Mini-Cog and Memory Impairment Screen are each simple quick preliminary screening tools, take less than 3 minutes to complete, and can be administered by trained office staff.[10,11]

EVALUATION

When there is concern about cognitive impairment, whether by patient or family complaint or screening, further evaluation is warranted. There are a variety of possible causes for cognitive impairment in an older adult that must be considered:

- Medication side effects
- Metabolic or endocrine problems
- Depression
- Delirium caused by illness (eg, pneumonia, urinary tract infection)
- Dementia.

There is general agreement about the basic components of the evaluation of cognitive impairment (**Box 2**). The first goal is to identify conditions that are treatable that may be causing or contributing to cognitive decline. This starts with a history from the patient about what they have been experiencing. Often, patients are not aware of their cognitive deficits or, owing to recent short-term memory problems, cannot recall and report difficulties. A family member or other knowledgeable informant who can corroborate and provide additional information about the patient's cognitive abilities and function should be interviewed as part of the evaluation.

An essential component of the evaluation of an older adult with changes in cognitive ability is an assessment of function. Early signs of cognitive difficulties that are often missed or ignored by patients, family, and providers include tasks that require attention, judgment, and reasoning; as well as those that involve multitasking. These include medication management, banking, finances, paying bills, and driving. Asking specifically about problems in these areas may provide clues to early cognitive decline. The short version of the Informant Questionnaire on Cognitive Decline in the Elderly (IQCODE) has been found to be easy to use and interpret with community-dwelling older adults.[12]

Box 1
Questions to detect cognitive impairment

1. During the past 12 months have you experienced confusion or memory loss that is happening more often or getting worse?

2. During the past 7 days, did you need help from others to perform everyday activities such as eating, getting dressed, grooming, bathing, walking, or using the toilet?

3. During the past 7 days, did you need help from others to take care of things such as laundry and housekeeping, banking, shopping, using the telephone, food preparation, transportation, or taking your own medication?

Box 2
Steps of basic evaluation of cognitive impairment

1. Interview patient and informant: memory or cognition, mood, behavior, function

2. Medication review: prescribed, over-the-counter, or recreational that cross blood–brain barrier

3. Physical examination: mental status screening, depression screening, cardiovascular and neurologic examination

4. Laboratory: complete blood count, chemistry panel, thyroid stimulating hormone, Vitamin B12, syphilis serology

5. Imaging: computed tomography or MRI brain

A thorough review of medications, prescribed and over-the-counter (OTC), is essential, with a focus on identification of pharmacologic agents that can contribute to cognitive dysfunction. Major classes of prescribed agents that are known to slow brain function and can cause or contribute to cognitive impairment in older adults are

- Benzodiazepines
- Sedative hypnotics
- Antipsychotics
- Anticholinergics
- Opiates.

Discontinuation of many of the medications in these classes should not be done abruptly. Deprescribing by slow taper of the medication over weeks or sometimes months is required, depending on the dosage and the length of time used. The antihistamine diphenhydramine, which is in many OTC products for sleep, is a common culprit contributing or causing cognitive impairment in the elderly. Additionally, alcohol use, as well as recreational drug use, must be investigated and should be discontinued whenever there is question of cognitive impairment.

An essential component of the evaluation of cognitive impairment is mental status testing. Many tools for clinical use are available that are easy to administer and score, with results that can be easily interpreted by a medical provider. Some of the most commonly used are listed in **Box 3**. The Mini-Mental State Examination (MMSE), once the gold standard, has fallen out of favor. It is now proprietary, was designed for detection of dementia, and is not valid for early detection.[13,14] The Montreal Cognitive Assessment (MoCA) is designed for detection of early cognitive changes in the clinical setting.[15] It is available in multiple languages, with several versions in some languages, which makes it useful with a variety of populations. The Modified MMSE

Box 3
Commonly used mental status screening tools

Mini-Mental State Examination (MMSE)

Montreal Cognitive Assessment (MoCA)

Modified Mini-Mental State Examination (3MS)

St. Louis University Mental Status Examination (SLUMS)

Geriatric Practitioner Assessment of Cognition Screening Test (GPCoG)

(3MS) is an expanded version of the MMSE that is available in English and Spanish that has components missing in the MMSE, which improves its usefulness in detection.[16] The St. Louis University Mental Status (SLUMS) Examination, also available in multiple languages, and the General Practitioner Assessment of Cognition (GPCoG) instrument are other commonly used instruments in primary care.[17,18]

Depression screening is critically important. Depression can both cause cognitive impairment and is a common symptom among older adults with MCI or early dementia. The short version of the Geriatric Depression Scale (GDS) is a brief questionnaire that is designed to assess for depression in older adults.[19] More general depression screening tools, such as the Patient Health Questionnaire (PHQ)-9, can be used but have not been specifically validated in older adults.

A physical examination with focus on the cardiovascular and neurologic examinations is essential. Abnormalities in cardiac function, such as arrhythmia or heart failure, can affect cognitive function. Neurologic examination may demonstrate subtle signs of a possible stroke, parkinsonism, or other neurologic condition that can contribute to or cause cognitive dysfunction.

Laboratory testing is done primarily to identify contributing or reversible causes. A complete blood count will identify anemias, as well as occasional other hematologic abnormalities that can contribute to slowed cognitive function. An elevated white count or, more commonly, a left shift, should signal the need to look for an underlying infection. Serum chemistry is important to identify hepatic or renal insufficiency. Thyroid stimulating hormone level is used to screen for hypothyroid and hyperthyroid, both conditions that occur with increased frequency in older adults and have associated cognitive changes. Vitamin B-12, essential for nerve function, is poorly absorbed with increasing age, and can be associated with both peripheral neuropathy and cognitive changes. There is some controversy about the role of syphilis screening in all patients with cognitive decline but it is still frequently recommended. Additional laboratory tests that should be considered in the evaluation of some older patients based on history or examination findings are sedimentation rate, methylmalonic acid, human immunodeficiency virus, and (if vasculitis is suspected) double-stranded DNA.

Brain imaging with computed tomography or MRI has primarily been used to rule out an underlying stroke, tumor, or other intracerebral abnormality, such as normal pressure hydrocephalus (NPH). NPH is a treatable and potentially reversible cause of cognitive decline associated with changes in gait and urinary incontinence, both very common coexisting findings in older adults.

DIAGNOSIS

Distinguishing between normal cognitive changes with age and decline that is indicative of indicates more serious underlying neurodegenerative disease remains challenging. Increased understanding of the pathologic changes that lead to Alzheimer disease and other dementing illnesses has required changes in terminology to reflect a spectrum of cognitive change that may occur, more commonly in older adults. Improvement in recognition of subtle changes in cognitive function (eg, memory, language, judgment, reasoning, visuospatial skills) that are not associated with a change in function and do not interfere with usual activities is categorized as mild cognitive impairment (MCI). In about half of patients diagnosed with MCI, this may represent very early signs of dementia but in other older adults the changes experienced persist but do not progress. The presence of cognitive decline, usually involving recent or short-term memory and other areas of cognition associated with a change in function, is considered to be a dementia syndrome. Revised terminology in the *Diagnostic and*

Statistical Manual of Mental Disorders, fifth edition, redefines dementia as a "major neurocognitive disorder" and considers MCI a "minor neurocognitive disorder."[20]

The most common underlying cause of dementia in older adults is Alzheimer disease. Late-onset Alzheimer disease (LOAD), which accounts for approximately 60% of dementias in the older population, is defined as the onset of Alzheimer disease after the age 65 years. The diagnosis of LOAD has been mainly based on exclusion using the workup previously outlined. Changes on a brain MRI of generalized atrophy and, specifically, hippocampal atrophy are nonspecific but highly suggestive of an underlying Alzheimer pathologic condition. Additionally, a fluorodeoxyglucose (FDG)-PET scan may show a pattern of decreased glucose uptake that is consistent with Alzheimer disease.

Several biomarkers have been developed to aid in differentiating the underlying pathologic condition and increase accurate diagnosis of Alzheimer disease. A PET scan using an amyloid tracer, approved by the FDA, can demonstrate the underlying amyloid pathologic condition in the brain; however, it is currently not reimbursed by Medicare or any other insurance carrier. Tests of cerebrospinal fluid that assess the presence of the 2 proteins associated with the development of neurofibrillary tangles (tau) and plaques (amyloid) are now available but remain expensive and are generally reserved for unusual cases or research.

Other less common causes of dementia in older adults usually have associated abnormal findings in the history or physical examination that can point the primary care provider away from Alzheimer disease. Patients with Lewy body disease may have rapid eye movement (REM) sleep disorder, visual hallucinations, parkinsonism on physical examination, and cognitive impairment with memory less severely impaired. Patients with an underlying vascular pathologic condition usually have vascular risk factors (eg, hypertension, diabetes, coronary artery disease, hyperlipidemia) and may have silent strokes or other changes on brain imaging to suggest this underlying etiologic factor. Frontotemporal lobar degeneration has several variants, presents with marked expressive language difficulty (semantic variant or primary progressive aphasia) or marked behavioral changes (severe apathy, sexual disinhibition, impulsivity), and an MRI shows atrophy of the frontal and temporal lobes with paring of the parietal lobes.

REFERRAL

Referral to a neuropsychologist for comprehensive neuropsychological testing can be extremely useful when mental status screening test results are normal and no other identifiable cause is found in a thorough evaluation. This testing can take several hours and help to uncover subtle areas of cognitive deficit that may be missed, especially in highly educated individuals. It can also pick up deficits in areas that are not assessed in the screening instrument.

The basic evaluation of memory complaints or other cognitive change and a diagnosis of typical LOAD is within the scope of primary care practice.[21] The decision of whether to refer to a specialist, such as a geriatrician, neurologist, geriatric psychiatrist, or memory disorders center, will depend on the primary care provider's experience and expertise. It will also depend on what resources are available in the community and, increasingly, on health system protocols. Patients with abnormal neurologic examination findings such as parkinsonism or deficits suggestive of underlying cerebrovascular disease should be referred to a neurologist. When behavior abnormalities are prominent, consideration of referral to a psychiatrist is appropriate. Complex patients with dementia and multiple comorbidities may be best managed by a geriatric specialist or geriatric team, if available.

After cognitive impairment has been identified and confirmed through an appropriate evaluation and a diagnosis is made, the focus shifts to ongoing management. A meeting with the patient and family members and others who are close the patient is recommended for discussion of the diagnosis and its implication for current and future care needs. In addition to ongoing medical management either by primary care or a specialist, referrals to the local senior services agency, local Alzheimer organization, or other community resources is important because many of the care needs are nonmedical. Provider or clinical practice identification of and referral to a single key agency, social worker, or geriatric care manager to assist patients with cognitive impairment or dementia diagnosis can make ongoing care easier for everyone.

REFERENCES

1. Alzheimers Association. Latest facts and figures report 2017. https://www.alz.org/facts/. Accessed Feburary 5, 2018.
2. Heron M. Death: leading causes for 2014. National vital statistics report, Vol. 65(5). Hyattsville (MD): National Center for Health Statistics; 2016.
3. Boustani M, Peterson D, Harris R, et al. Screening for dementia. Rockville (MD): Agency for Healthcare Research and Quality; 2003. Available at: http//:www.ncbi.nim.nh.gov/books/NBK42773/.
4. Chodosh J, Petitti DB, Elliott M, et al. Physician recognition of cognitive impairment: evaluating the need for improvement. J Am Geriatr Soc 2004;52:1051–9.
5. Kotagai V, Langa KM, Plassman BL, et al. Factors associated with cognitive evaluations in the United States. Neurology 2015;84(1):64–71.
6. NIA assessing cognitive impairment in older patients.
7. Medicare coverage of Annual Wellness visit providing a personalized prevention plan. Fed Regist 2010;75:73401.
8. Behavioral risk factor surveillance system survey questionnaire. Bethesda (MD): Centers for Diseae Control and Prevention. Available at: http://www.cdc.gov/brfss/questionnaires/pdf-ques/2011brfss.pdf.
9. Galvin JE, Roe CM, Powlishta KK, et al. The AD8: a brief informant interview to detect dementia. Neurology 2005;65(4):559–64.
10. Borson S, Scanlan J, Brush M, et al. The Mini-Cog: a cognitive 'vital signs' measure for dementia screening in multi-lingual elderly. Int J Geriatr Psychiatry 2000; 15(11):1021–7.
11. Buschke H, Kuslansky G, Katz M, et al. Screening for dementia with the memory impairment screen. Neurology 1999;52(2):231–8.
12. Quinn TJ, Fearon P, Noell-Storr AH. The Informant Questionnaire on Cognitive Impairment in the Elderly (IQCODE) for the diagnosis of dementia in community dwelling populations. Cochrane Database Syst Rev 2014;(4):CD010079.
13. Folstein M, Folstein S, McHugh P. Mini-mental state; a practical method for grading cognitive state of patients for clinicians. J Psychiatr Res 1975;12(3): 189–98.
14. Trenkle D, Shankle R, Azen S. Detecting cognitive impairment in primary care: performance assessment of three screening instruments. J Alzheimers Dis 2007;11(3):323–35.
15. Nasreddine ZA, Phillips NA, Bedrian V, et al. The Montreal Cognitive Assessment, MoCA; a brief screening tool for mild cognitive impairment. J Am Geriatr Soc 2005;53(4):695–9.
16. Teng E, Chui H. The Modified Mini-Mental State (3MS) examination. J Clin Psychiatry 1987;48:314–8.

17. St Louis University Mental State (SLUMS) Examination. Available at: https://www.slu.edu/medicine/internal-medicine/geriatric-medicine/aging-sucessfully/assessment-tools/mental-status-exam.php.
18. Brodaty H, Pond D, Kemp NM, et al. The GPCOG: a new screening test for dementia designed for general practice. J Am Geriatr Soc 2002;50:530–4.
19. Sheikh JI, Yesavage JA. Geriatric Depression Scale (GDS): recent evidence and development of a shorter version. Clinc Gerontol: The J Aging and Mentl Health 1986;5(1–2):165–73.
20. American Psychiatric Association. Diagnostic and statistical manual of mental disorders. 5th edition. 2013.
21. Galvin JE, Sadowsky CH. Practical guidelines for the recognition and diagnosis of dementia. J Am Board Fam Med 2012;25:367–82.

Advance Care Planning
Advance Directives and Physician Orders for Life-Sustaining Treatment

Judy Thomas, JD[a], Amy Vandenbroucke, JD[b], Kelley Queale, BA[a],*

KEYWORDS

- Advance care planning • Advance directive
- Physician orders for life-sustaining treatment • POLST • End of life

KEY POINTS

- Advance care planning (ACP) is a process that supports adults at any age or stage of health in understanding and sharing their personal values, life goals, and preferences regarding future medical care.
- ACP increases the likelihood that an individual's treatment wishes will be known and respected during serious illness and at the end of life.
- Communication between individuals, family, and health care providers is the cornerstone of ACP.
- Completion of an ACP form, such as an advance directive or physician order for life-sustaining treatment, is just a single element of the ACP process.
- The primary goal of ACP is ensuring that individuals receive medical treatment that is consistent with their values, goals, and preferences during serious illness or at the end of life.

INTRODUCTION

Advance care planning (ACP) is a multistep process that involves an ongoing dialogue between individuals and health care providers in which individuals are supported in (1) understanding treatment options for end-of-life care in the context of their own medical conditions; (2) exploring their personal values and beliefs regarding end-of-life care; and (3) sharing their wishes regarding future medical care and treatment with family, surrogates, and physicians. This article offers an overview of ACP and its benefits to individuals and providers. ACP forms, such as advance directives (ADs) and physician orders for life-sustaining treatment (POLST) are defined, compared, and contrasted.

[a] Coalition for Compassionate Care of California, 1331 Garden Highway, Suite 100, Sacramento, CA 95833, USA; [b] National POLST Paradigm, 208 I Street Northeast, Washington, DC 20002, USA
* Corresponding author.
E-mail address: kqueale@CoalitionCCC.org

Physician Assist Clin 3 (2018) 495–503
https://doi.org/10.1016/j.cpha.2018.05.004
2405-7991/18/© 2018 Elsevier Inc. All rights reserved.

physicianassistant.theclinics.com

ADVANCE CARE PLANNING

ACP is a process that supports adults at any age or stage of health in understanding and sharing their personal values, life goals, and preferences regarding future medical care. The goal of ACP is to help ensure that people receive medical care that is consistent with their values, goals, and preferences during serious and chronic illness.[1]

When asked about end-of-life treatment wishes, most people indicate they would prefer to die at home instead of in a hospital or nursing home, and they would rather focus on quality of life rather than extending their life through all possible medical interventions. Also, most people say that they want to talk to their health care team about their goals and wishes for treatment at end of life.[2]

Unfortunately, despite passage in 1990 of the Patient Self-Determination Act,[3] which requires most institutional providers and health maintenance organizations that participate in Medicare or Medicaid to implement programs that inform patients about their rights to make medical decisions, ACP conversations are not happening as routinely as recommended.

Benefits of Advance Care Planning

ACP increases the likelihood that an individual's treatment wishes will be known and respected during serious illness and at the end of life, making it an integral part of patient-centered care. Individuals who engage in ACP stand to gain

- A better sense of control over their future health care
- Improved outcomes and quality of life
- Increased likelihood that they will die in their preferred setting
- Stronger relationships with their health providers and loved ones through open communication
- Peace of mind in knowing that loved ones are relieved of the burden of guessing about their wishes during a medical crisis.

Providers also realize valuable benefits when patients' health care wishes are solicited, recorded, and honored, including

- Avoiding over-treating or under-treating patients, allowing for more efficient use of care resources
- Improved communication between patients and providers
- Increased use of hospice and palliative care
- Reduced rates of rehospitalization at the end of life.

Conversations Around Advance Care Planning

ACP is not a single discussion but a continual conversation over time as an individual's health condition and goals of medical treatment change (**Fig. 1**). Because a medical crisis can happen at any age or any stage of a person's life, the ACP process ideally begins at age 18 years. When end-of-life goals and treatment options are explored earlier in the disease process, individuals and their families have more time to choose the path that best fits their needs.[4,5]

Ideally, the ACP process involves multiple, in-depth conversations between the individual, family members, and providers, which are conducted at various stages of the person's life. Conversations about treatment goals and health status are conducted by the physician; however, other members of the health care team can and should play an important role in ACP. For example, the specialized training and communications skills of physician assistants (PAs), advanced practice nurses (APNs), and social workers make them particularly well-suited to be a part of the ACP team.

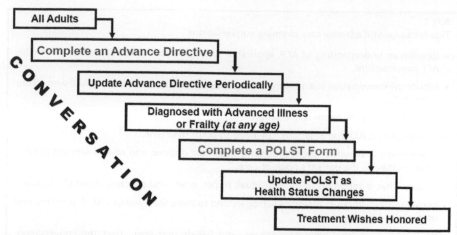

Fig. 1. ADs and POLST. (*Courtesy of* the Coalition for Compassionate Care of California, Sacramento, CA, CoalitionCCC.org.)

Recognizing the importance and benefit of ACP conversations, the Centers for Medicare & Medicaid Services (CMS) issued a final rule activating 2 ACP codes (99497 and 99498) as part of its 2016 Medicare physician fee schedule. Medicare now covers ACP as a separate service by providers who bill CMS using the physician fee schedule. Some state Medicaid programs and private insurers have since followed Medicare's lead and provide reimbursement of ACP conversations with beneficiaries.

Cultural Complexities

Though it can be helpful to know in general how different groups may respond to issues related to death and dying, that knowledge is best used as a starting point for approaching ACP conversations, not as a way of categorizing individuals. Sensitivity to ethnic and cultural diversity may unwittingly lead to unsubstantiated assumptions about individuals and population groups. Just as those within a family who are raised with similar beliefs and backgrounds can have very different views on any given subject, so may those who share a common cultural background. See **Box 1** for more tips for successful ACP conversations.

Advance Care Planning Tools and Resources

There are many resources to help individuals, families, and providers have ACP conversations and document treatment wishes. Some resources to consider include

- The Conversation Project's starter kit has multiple versions. All are intended to help people have conversations with their family members or other loved ones about their wishes regarding end-of-life care; materials are available in several languages. They also have tools called "How to Choose a Health Care Proxy" and "How to Be a Health Care Proxy."
- The American Bar Association's *Care Planning Toolkit* has 9 tools that help individuals clarify and communicate what is important to them through self-help worksheets, resources, and suggestions.
- The National POLST Paradigm provides information on POLST, links to state POLST programs, and resources for providers and consumers.

> **Box 1**
> **Tips for successful advance care planning conversations**
>
> - Develop an understanding of ACP, applicable state laws, forms, and elements of effective ACP conversations.
> - Initiate the conversation in a nonthreatening manner, "We like to talk about ACP with all our patients."
> - Allow time for an in-depth conversation.
> - Recognize that ACP conversations may need to occur over time.
> - Give realistic information about prognosis, treatment options, and what treatment options mean relative to the patient's goals of care.
> - Explore what is important to the individual: hopes, goals, and concerns about the future.
> - Encourage individuals to identify a surrogate and to share their wishes with that person and others who are close.
> - Be aware of personal attitudes, culture, and beliefs that may affect the conversation, including those of providers.

- The Coalition for Compassionate Care of California provides free and low-cost resources and videos related to ACP and palliative care.
- PREPARE, also referred to as PREPARE for Your Care, is an interactive Web site serving as a resource for families navigating medical decision-making.
- The GoWish Game can be played with cards or online and is a simple way to think and talk about what's important to individuals and their family members if someone becomes seriously ill.
- Heart to Heart cards is a bilingual (Chinese or English) communication activity designed to make it easier to understand what people might prefer when their lives are threatened by injury or disease.
- Hello (formerly The Gift of Grace) is a conversation game to help individuals identify their values and what makes a good quality of life.
- National Healthcare Decisions Day (April 16th) provides an opportunity and resources for organizations, facilities, and individuals to promote ACP.

Documenting the Conversation

Documentation of ACP conversations can take several forms. The most common include

- Durable power of attorney or health care proxy. This is a legal document in which the patient appoints a trusted agent or proxy to make medical decisions on her or his behalf in the event the patient loses capacity.
- Living will. This is a written, legal document in which the patient outlines the types of life-sustaining treatments she or he wants or does not want if the patient has a terminal illness or is in a persistent vegetative state.
- Advance Directive (AD). Some states combine the durable power of attorney and living will into a single document, called an AD.
- POLST. Some states call this Medical Orders for Life-Sustaining Treatment or similar names. The POLST form is a medical order for the specific medical treatments a patient wants during a medical emergency. POLST forms are appropriate for individuals with a serious illness or advanced frailty near the end of life.
- Progress notes or chart notes. The conversation may also be recorded as notes in an individual's medical record.

ADs and POLST forms are both called ACP documents; however, they are not the same. An AD is a legal document and the POLST form is a medical order.

PHYSICIAN ORDERS FOR LIFE-SUSTAINING TREATMENT

Although all competent adults, regardless of health status, should have an AD, the POLST form is only appropriate for those who are seriously ill or frail, whose medical provider would not be surprised if the individual died within a year. A key difference between them is that emergency medical personnel can provide the treatment options identified on the POLST form because it is a medical order. **Table 1** provides further distinctions.

Emergency personnel are required by law to do everything possible to attempt to save someone's life absent a medical order to the contrary. If a patient only has an AD, life-saving treatment will be attempted, and the person will be transported to the hospital, where the hospital's health care team will work with the surrogate identified in the AD to review the individual's wishes and develop a treatment plan.

As a medical order, the POLST form directs emergency personnel about what treatment (eg, advanced airway interventions) to provide during an emergency, helping ensure the individual only receives transportation to the hospital and treatment (eg, mechanical ventilation or manual treatment of airway obstruction) that matches their wishes.

Importantly, ADs and POLST forms can be revoked orally or in writing by a patient with capacity at any time.

ADs and POLST can and should work together. An AD provides guidance on health care decision-making from age 18 years through death. When an individual becomes seriously ill or frail, the use of a POLST form becomes appropriate. An existing AD may

Table 1
How is an advance directive different from a physician order for life-sustaining treatment?

	POLST Paradigm Form	Advance Directive
Type of Document	Medical order	Legal document
Who Completes?	Health care professional (and patient or surrogate)	Individual
Who Needs a POLST?	Seriously ill or frail (any age) patient for whom health care professional would not be surprised if died within year	All competent adults
Appoints a Surrogate?	No	Yes
What is Communicated?	Specific medical orders for treatment wishes during a medical emergency	General wishes about treatment wishes May help guide treatment plan after a medical emergency
Can Emergency Medical Services Use?	Yes	No
Ease in Locating	Very easy to find Patient has original Copy is in medical record Copy may be in registry (if your state has a registry)	Not very easy to find Depends on where patient keeps it and if they have told someone where it is, or given a copy to surrogate or to health professional to put in his or her medical record

National POLST Paradigm January 2018.

help shape the individual's treatment choices when discussing POLST form options with their provider.

History and Development

The POLST Paradigm started in 1991 when leading medical ethicists in Oregon discovered that individual preferences for end-of-life care were not consistently being honored. Recognizing that ADs were inadequate for individuals with serious illness or frailty (who frequently require emergency medical care), a group of stakeholders developed a new tool for honoring individuals' wishes for end-of-life treatment. After several years of evaluation, the program became known as POLST.

The POLST movement then spread to other states, initially New York, Pennsylvania, Washington, West Virginia, and Wisconsin, which renamed, adapted and implemented POLST Paradigm initiatives to fit their states' own cultural and legislative cultures. Leaders from these states and Oregon formed what became the National POLST Paradigm Task Force, which sets quality standards for POLST forms and programs and assists states in developing POLST programs. It set up a national office at the Oregon Health and Science University's Center for Ethics in Health Care to manage outreach, education, policy development, and research; to support implementation efforts in other states; and to disseminate lessons learned. The National Office continues these activities as part of the Tides Center.

Currently, all 50 states and Washington, DC, have taken steps to implement the POLST Paradigm; 22 states are endorsed, meaning that the Task Force confirmed their form and the program complies with endorsement standards. As a note, POLST is the generic identifier for all programs fitting its definition regardless of the actual term used in a state; individual terms for states can be found on the POLST Paradigm map.

How the Paradigm Works

The POLST Paradigm is an approach to end-of-life planning that helps elicit, document, and honor individual treatment wishes for seriously ill or frail individuals through conversations and use of a portable out-of-hospital or facility medical order that is intended to accompany an individual on transitions across care settings, including in the home.

The POLST Paradigm is intended to be used by individuals who are seriously ill or frail, and whose providers would not be surprised if they died within a year (regardless of age or care setting). Care setting or age is not a reliable trigger for POLST. For example, an individual admitted to a skilled nursing facility for short-term rehabilitation following hip surgery may not be appropriate for POLST, whereas a 22-year old with kidney disease might be.

Just as individuals may choose to refuse treatment or not to have an AD, individuals may decline to complete a POLST. Similarly, completion of a POLST form without the knowledge of the patient or surrogate is contrary to the purpose and intent of the POLST Paradigm and violates informed consent and principles of person-centered and family-centered care.[6]

Elements of the Form

Although the layout and text of POLST forms may vary by state, specific form elements are required for programs that are endorsed by the POLST Task Force. For example, in Section B (the medical intervention section), some states list the treatment options from most aggressive to least aggressive, whereas others begin with the least aggressive. Substantively, however, they are the same. Side 1 of the POLST form provides the medical orders and consists of at least 3 sections:

- Section A is about cardiopulmonary resuscitation (CPR) wishes. This section only applies when the individual is unresponsive, has no pulse, and is not breathing; this section does not apply to any other medical circumstance. The POLST form goes beyond a do-not-resuscitate order by allowing individuals to affirmatively state that they want CPR attempted.
- Section B, the heart of the POLST form, provides the medical interventions the individual wants during a medical emergency when she or he cannot communicate but CPR is not appropriate. When the question of CPR is irrelevant, this section guides emergency personnel in deciding what treatment to provide and whether to transport the individual to the hospital. Three options are provided along with space for the provider to write in orders specific to the individual. POLST forms are only about treatment options; care is always provided. There are 3 options:
  1. Full treatment. The goal of this option is to prolong life by all medically effective means. The individual may receive potentially life-sustaining treatments, including intubation, advanced airway intervention, mechanical ventilation, cardioversion, transfer to the hospital, and intensive care, as indicated, with no limitation of treatment. In many states, choosing CPR in Section A requires choosing full treatment in Section B.
  2. Limited treatment or selective treatment. The goal is to provide individuals with basic medical treatments while avoiding burdensome measures. The individual will be hospitalized if necessary; however, mechanical ventilation and intensive care unit treatments will be avoided. This option is appropriate for individuals whose goal is to obtain treatments for reversible conditions or exacerbations of the underlying disease with the goal of restoring the individual to his or her current state of health.
  3. Comfort measures only. The goal is to maximize comfort through symptom management and may include use of antibiotics (some states have antibiotics as a separate section on the POLST form). Individuals choosing this option want to avoid hospitalizations unless necessary to ensure comfort needs are met.
- Section C discusses artificially administered nutrition and hydration. All POLST forms state that fluids and nutrition will be offered if medically feasible.

The bottom part of a POLST form includes 2 additional sections: conversation information and signatures. The conversation information documents who was involved in the conversation leading up to the completion of the POLST form. Forms may provide checkboxes, showing the conversation occurred with the individual or surrogate, or that it was based on the individual's AD.

Side 2 of a POLST form has directions and information, usually for providers, such as how to complete, update, and void a POLST form. It may also include contact information for surrogates and information on providers or interpreters who assisted in completing the POLST form.

Conversations

Conversations between the provider and patient or surrogate are crucial to the completion of a POLST form. POLST form completion is a single step in a process that includes and, in fact, depends on conversations around the individual's current diagnosis, prognosis, treatment options (including risks and benefits of each), and goals of care. A conversation may result in a completed POLST form or it may just be a first step in the care planning process.

The POLST form uses medical terms that not all individuals understand. Therefore, it is important that treatment options are shared using language and tools (eg, videos or visuals) that assist individuals and families in developing a clear understanding of the information.

The Task Force recommends that physicians, APNs, and PAs be permitted to participate in the POLST Paradigm process and to sign POLST forms. The Task Force also strongly encourages training of all providers who complete POLST forms. For example, the Coalition for Compassionate Care of California developed a specialized POLST curriculum and program that has trained more than 1000 providers over the past several years.

Because the POLST form is a medical order, a licensed health care provider is required to sign the form for it to be valid, although which providers may sign varies by state. All states with POLST programs authorize physicians (doctors of medicine and doctors of osteopathic medicine) to sign POLST forms. An increasing number now also authorize PAs, APNs, and naturopaths to sign based on their education, training, and practice abilities.

Because POLST forms are medical orders completed by providers to communicate treatment decisions to other providers, it is never appropriate to provide a POLST form to an individual, surrogate, or family member to complete independently.

The National POLST Paradigm strongly recommends, and most states require, that the patient (or surrogate) also sign the form to demonstrate that the individual or surrogate was part of the conversation.

Keeping the Form Current

It is critical that a patient's POLST form be reviewed periodically to ensure that the medical orders match the current treatment plan and individual treatment wishes. In its legislative guide, the Task Force recommends POLST forms be reviewed when the individual is transferred between care settings or care levels; when there is a substantial change in the individual's health status; or when the individual's goals of care, treatment preferences, or both change.

Portability

The POLST form is designed to travel with the patient in the community and across care settings. To ease patient burden and facilitate emergency personnel locating POLST forms immediately when necessary, some states are turning to electronic POLST registries.

Electronic registries allow for the secure storage of POLST information that can be immediately located and accessed by authorized medical providers, including emergency responders in the field. Emergency personnel in Oregon, for example, are trained to call the Oregon POLST Registry anytime (1) they suspect a patient has a POLST form, (2) they are told a patient has a POLST form but are unable to locate it, (3) the patient has a chronic progressive illness, (4) the patient is frail or elderly, or (5) a POLST form is produced on the scene but there is a problem or question about the orders selected or validity of the form.

Electronic registries remove responsibility from individuals by eliminating the need for the seriously ill or frail individual to remember to bring the form with them at all appointments, to carry the POLST form with them at all times, and to remember to place the form in a location that emergency personnel are trained to look. A centralized registry may also help ensure that all providers across a region or state have access to a patient's most current POLST form orders.

Currently, only a handful of states (Oregon, Idaho, Washington, West Virginia, and New York) are operating fully functional statewide registries. Other states, such as

California, are currently pilot testing local POLST registries with a goal of future state-wide implementation.

Technology and the Paradigm

In addition to improving provider access to completed POLST forms across large communities, technology is being harnessed to improve access to POLST orders within organizations, eliminate form completion errors, and streamline administrative components of the form. For example, electronic medical records (EMR) can be designed to flag patient records containing POLST orders and make the information immediately accessible with a single click. When POLST forms are completed using e-form technology linked to the EMR, time can be saved and errors eliminated through auto-filling of individual demographics and provider information (name, license number, date of signature). Additionally, e-forms can be programmed to prevent the creation of POLST with incompatible order sets, such as CPR and comfort measures only. The potential also exists to ensure any other orders entered in an individual's EMR are consistent with POLST form orders. Finally, it helps ensure POLST orders are immediately available; the Task Force encourages all facilities to set up their EMRs to keep POLST orders in a single location immediately accessible with a single click.

Integration of POLST forms within EHRs is slowly increasing; however, health care systems are often challenged by the lack of related best practices and guidance, as well as issues with interoperability.

SUMMARY

When individuals are in the midst of a medical crisis or nearing the end of life, they are often physically or mentally incapable of making their own health care decisions. Family members and health care providers need clear guidance from the patient to ensure that the medical treatment provided fully aligns with the patient's wishes, goals, and values. ACP fills an important role in patient-centered care, by helping individuals explore their wishes in the context of their medical condition, values, and beliefs, and share those wishes with family, surrogates and physicians. Successful ACP programs are incorporated into routine care because ACP is not a 1-time act but an ongoing conversation that is best revisited over the course of a lifetime.

REFERENCES

1. Sudore RL, Lum HD, You JJ, et al. Defining advance care planning for adults: a consensus definition from a multidisciplinary Delphi panel. J Pain Symptom Manage 2017;53:821.
2. Lake Partners and CCCC. Final chapter: Californians' attitudes and experiences with death and dying. California Health Care Foundation; 2012. Available at: http://www.chcf.org/publications/2012/02/final-chapter-death-dying.
3. H.R. 5835 — 101st Congress: Omnibus Budget Reconciliation Act of 1990. Available at: https://www.govtrack.us/congress/bills/101/hr5835. Accessed June 21, 2018.
4. Ferrell BR. Late referrals to palliative care. J Clin Oncol 2005;23(12):2588–9.
5. National Hospice and Palliative Care Organization. NHPCO facts and figures: hospice care in America. Alexandria (VA): National Hospice and Palliative Care Organization; 2009.
6. National POLST Paradigm, Appropriate POLST paradigm form use policy. Available at: http://polst.org/wp-content/uploads/2017/05/2017.05.18-Appropriate-POLST-Paradigm-Form-Use-Policy.pdf. Accessed January 22, 2018.

Palliative Care of the Older Adult

Richard J. Ackermann, MD[a,b,]*, Rosegenee Ellis, MD[c]

KEYWORDS

- Palliative care • Hospice • Communication • Nonpain symptoms • Family meetings
- Artificial hydration and nutrition

KEY POINTS

- Palliative care is an interdisciplinary focus on improving quality of life for patients who suffer from severe chronic or terminal illness, whereas hospice is a model of care that focuses on patients with a life expectancy of less than 6 months.
- Older adults with decision-making capacity are awake and able to receive information, understand the risks and benefits or proposed alternatives, and can articulate a treatment preference.
- Dyspnea is a subjective sensation of breathlessness that differs from patient to patient. At the end of life, dyspnea may respond to air directed at the face, low-dose opioids, a benzodiazepine, or oxygen.
- At the end of life, respiratory secretions are generally more distressing to the family than to the patient. Because muscarinic antagonists have limited effectiveness and substantial adverse effects, nonpharmacologic treatments, such as stopping intravenous hydration, positioning, and reducing the frequency of turning, should be the first steps.
- Physician assistants should feel confident recommending against tube feeding in patients with advanced dementia. This intervention has no benefit in preventing pneumonia or pressure sores, does not enhance survival, and medicalizes the end of life.

INTRODUCTION

Among deaths in the United States, 85% occur in patients over 60 years old, with a median age of death of 77 years. Rather than dying suddenly, most older adults accumulate multiple chronic diseases that lead to progressive disability, dependence on others, and hospitalization. Goals of care usually change during this transition, progressing from a desire for aggressive curative treatment to a care strategy that values quality of life and comfort.[1] Compared with younger patients, older adults are more

Disclosure Statement: The authors having nothing to disclose.
[a] Hospice and Palliative Medicine Fellowship, Medical Center Navicent Health, 3780 Eisenhower Parkway, Macon, GA 31206, USA; [b] Department of Family Medicine, Mercer University School of Medicine, 1501 Mercer University Drive, Macon, GA 31207, USA; [c] Palliative Care Service, Medical Center Navicent Health, 777 Hemlock Street, Macon, GA 31210, USA
* Corresponding author. 3780 Eisenhower Parkway, Macon, GA 31206.
E-mail address: Ackermann.Richard@NavicentHealth.org

likely to have cognitive impairment, desire fewer interventions at the end of life, and live in an institution. Physiologic reserves become depleted, so minor perturbations, such as hyponatremia, may cascade to catastrophic loss of function or death.[2]

This article provides the physician assistant (PA) with an overview of the differences between palliative care and hospice, tips on communicating with older adults and their families about serious chronic disease, management of nonpain symptoms, and advice on artificial nutrition and hydration (ANH) at the end of life.

WHAT IS PALLIATIVE CARE?

Palliative care is an interdisciplinary focus on improving quality of life for patients who suffer from severe chronic or terminal illness. Palliative care should be available from the time of diagnosis of a life-threatening illness and may be provided concurrently with curative or disease-modifying treatments.[3] The most common site for nonhospice palliative care is the hospital, with 75% of hospitals with more than 50 beds having a palliative service in 2015.[4] Randomized trials document that these programs improve symptoms, quality of life, and family satisfaction, and they reduce costs. Nearly all nursing homes have a relationship with hospice, and in some communities, palliative care consultation or a specialized unit is available in this setting.

An important goal of modern palliative care is to transform medicine from the old dichotomy between curative and palliative care into a more integrated model, where the 2 coexist through the illness. In most patients with chronic disease, there comes a time when palliative care becomes the predominant or exclusive concern. Palliative care is a health care strategy that offers seriously ill patients and their families a comprehensive package of care by a team of professionals with expertise in addressing the multiple, complex problems that arise in the advanced stages of disease. Palliative clinicians work to achieve comfort and a peaceful death by improving quality of life for both patient and family. Palliative care is for anyone who is seriously ill, at any age, and at any stage of illness.

On the other hand, hospice is a model of care that focuses on symptom management and supports patients with a life expectancy of 6 months or less. The 6-month prognosis is arbitrary but is part of the eligibility criteria for the Medicare Hospice Benefit (MHB). Hospice can also refer to a place of care, such as an inpatient hospice facility. Hospice is a part of palliative care.

Palliative care is provided mainly in 2 places—hospice and hospital palliative care services. **Table 1** summarizes some of the differences between them. Hospice patients must meet a 6-month prognosis, whereas palliative clinicians manage patients at any stage of an advanced illness. Reimbursement to hospice is through a specified benefit package, whereas hospital palliative care has no independent revenue stream. In most communities, patients may choose among several hospices, although there is almost always a single palliative service in a hospital. The focus of hospice is providing comprehensive care to patients at the end of life by opting out of standard medical care, whereas hospital palliative care may be provided concurrently with disease-modifying regimens over a longer period.[5]

PAs should be comfortable in both providing palliative care and recommending hospice to their patients. The MHB is available if a patient desires a palliative approach to the illness and if 2 physicians (the attending physician and the hospice medical director) certify that a patient's life expectancy is 6 months or less if the disease takes its expected course.[6] The initial hospice certification is for 90 days, followed by another 90-day certification, followed by a potentially unlimited number of 60-day certifications. **Box 1** provides assistance in deciding when to refer patients to hospice.

Table 1
Comparing hospice and hospital palliative care services

Characteristic	Hospice	Hospital Palliative Care
Population	Prognosis less than six months Patients with prognosis 6–12 mo should be educated about hospice	Patients at any stage of advanced or life-limiting illness
Sites of care	Home, nursing home, assisted living facility, hospital, free-standing inpatient hospice	Hospital, often in the intensive care unit Some have outpatient palliative services
Services	Pain/symptom management, psychosocial and spiritual support, care coordination Delivered by a team with physicians, nurses, social workers, aides, chaplain, counselors, and volunteers Medical equipment, medications, supplies bereavement support for 1 y after death	Services vary by program, from a single health care provider to an interdisciplinary team
Financing	Per diem payment for 4 levels of care – routine home care, continuous home care, general inpatient care, and respite care Contributions support not-for-profit hospices	Reimbursed through existing payment channels
Length of stay	Mean 2 mo, median <20 d	Varies, care often episodic
Choice	Usually multiple	Usually only one service, larger hospitals likely to have dedicated palliative services
Role of the primary care clinician	May continue to manage medical care, backed up by the hospice medical director	May request a consult from the palliative team hospitalists often manage inpatient care
Staffing	A hospice team of 30 patients may have 3 nurses, 1–2 aides, 1 social worker, and part-time chaplains, therapists, and volunteers Staff certification in palliative care is desirable	Ideally include physicians, nurses, social worker, perhaps a pharmacist, psychologist, other therapists Staff certification in palliative care is desirable
Key differences	Focus on caring for the patient and family at the end of life Patient opts out of regular Medicare coverage for the terminal illness	Focus on providing expert palliative care throughout the continuum of severe illness Can be delivered concurrently with curative or life-prolonging therapies

Adapted from Teno JM, Connor SR. Referring a patient and family to high-quality palliative care at the close of life: "We met a new personality with this level of compassion and empathy". JAMA 2009;301:651–9; with permission.

Once enrolled in hospice, an interdisciplinary team, including a physician, nurse, bereavement counselor, chaplain, social worker, and others, devise a comprehensive and individualized plan for each patient. Health care legislation passed in February 2018 includes PAs as clinicians who can now receive reimbursement through the MHB. Medicare

---

Box 1
Medicare general guideline for hospice eligibility

The patient should meet all the following criteria:

1. Life-limiting condition

2. Patient/family informed condition is life limiting

3. Patient/family elects palliative care

4. Documentation of clinical progression of disease
   Evidenced by
   - Serial physician assessment
   - Laboratory studies
   - Radiologic or other studies
   - Inpatient hospitalizations
   - Home health nursing assessment if patient home homebound
   There must be either a recent decline in function or impaired nutrition status.
   Functional decline can be documented by a decline in Karnofsky Performance Scale or by increasing dependence in ≥3 activities of daily living:
   - Bathing
   - Dressing
   - Feeding
   - Transfers
   - Continence of urine and stool
   - Ambulation to bathroom
   Impaired nutritional status can be documented by either
   - Unintentional, progressive weight loss ≥10% over the past 6 mo
   - Serum albumin <2.5 g/dL

---

and most commercial insurance cover the costs of care for the terminal illness, including medical equipment and medications, as well as grief counseling for the family.

Despite this comprehensive insurance coverage, hospice services are underused, with only 46% of dying Americans using hospice services in 2015.[7] Most patients receiving hospice receive that care in their homes (home hospice). Inpatient hospice is available for brief intensive management of uncontrolled symptoms and for respite care that provides short breaks for families. A physician or PA can remain as a patient's primary clinician while the patient receives hospice services and can continue to see the patient, billing Medicare as usual.

COMMUNICATING WITH OLDER ADULTS AND THEIR FAMILIES

The PA should determine whether a patient has decision-making capacity. This determination should be made by the treating clinician, not relying on other providers' assessments. Simple orientation questions do not suffice. Patients need to be awake and able to receive information regarding diagnosis, understand the risks and benefits of proposed alternatives, and express a treatment preference in their own words. Clinicians do not have to agree with a patient's decision.

If a patient lacks decision-making capacity, then a surrogate decision-maker must be identified. Although providers tend to believe whoever is at the bedside can make decisions for the patient, this is not always the case. State laws should be reviewed regarding legal next of kin and who may determine resuscitation status or consent for procedures.

Skillful family meetings are the cornerstone of high-quality end-of-life care for older adults. They provide the venue where complex decisions are made as well as where conflicts are resolved.[8–10] **Box 2** summarizes the key steps for a successful family

---

Box 2
Steps for a structured family meeting on end-of-life issues

Prepare—set the agenda, invite appropriate family and staff, have a brief premeeting, identify a setting, sit in the center of the group.

Introduce the participants and the purpose of the meeting.

Assess a family's understanding of the medical conditions, prognosis, and their preference for decision making.

Summarize and educate.

Explore what the patient is experiencing now, including suffering.

Ask what the patient would want under the circumstances.

Frame recommendations in the light of the goals of care, seeking either consent or assent.

Facilitate grieving.

Plan for a follow-up meeting.

Discuss, debrief, and document.

Data from Billings JA, Block SD. The end-of-life family meeting in intensive care part III: a guide for structured discussions. J Palliat Med 2011;14(9):1058–64.

---

meeting. Ideally older adults make their own decisions or have delineated preferences in an advance directive. In many cases, however, family members need to speak for a patient.

The clinician, which could be a PA, should come prepared. Is this meeting to identify the decision makers or to gain consent for a medical intervention, such as tube feeding? Someone should find a quiet, comfortable, and private setting and bring tissues; everyone should turn off cell phones and pagers. After introducing everyone and understanding each family member's relationship to the patient, a warning shot may be indicated to emphasize the gravity of the situation, such as "I'm sorry: I have some really bad news to share with you."

The team needs to hear the family's understanding of the patient's medical conditions and prognosis as well as how they like to make decisions. The family can spin out their story, at least for a while, even if this narrative seems tangential. If inaccurate or incomplete understanding arises, the PA can use more focused questions and explanations. Next steps include summarizing what they have said and confirming that it is correct. A description of the patient's medical conditions, without medical jargon (eg, "His liver is failing," not "The Model for End-Stage Liver Disease score is 24 and his hepatic encephalopathy is refractory") can correct misunderstandings and fill in gaps. Before sharing bad news, the clinician should ask permission to do so, addressing all emotions in the room. It is often best to use the "D" word: "Despite our best efforts, we expect your mother to die in the next couple weeks." Another strategy is using "I wish" statements, such as "I wish things were different" and "I wish I had better news for you."

There may be evidence that the patient is suffering. Mechanical intubation, feeding tubes, chest tubes, restraints, blood draws, turning, and wound care cause suffering and pain. Treatments amy be causing too much suffering to justify a brief survival or survival to a recovery with very low function. If this discussion leads to a decision to withhold or withdraw medical interventions, emphasize that the team will still care for the patient, aggressively minimizing pain and other symptoms.

Often there is uncertainty how to proceed. Using the principle of substituted judgment, the PA can ask family members what they think the patient would decide in the situation, if the patient could participate for just 5 minutes. Rather than asking the family, "What do you think we should do?" a better question is, "What decision do you think Dad would make in this situation?"

As diseases progress, goals of care change. For example, an older cancer patient may choose cure as the initial goal, but this often changes to control and finally to comfort. When the disease can no longer be controlled, a patient's primary goal may become living pain-free, achieving closure in personal issues, or staying at home surrounded by family and friends.

Once the overall goal of care has been established, the clinician can frame recommendations that honor this preference. Sometimes the best approach is to provide a trial of treatment for several days and reassess. In other cases, a clear recommendation to withdraw life support or access hospice can be made. Never speak the words, it is best to avoid saying "Do you want us to do everything?" because that places a large burden on family members, and the logical answer is, "Yes, of course, he's my father." When faced with life-threatening illness, many patients and clinicians believe they must choose between 2 extremes, either hoping for remission of the disease or preparing for death. One strategy is to embrace hope while also preparing for decline: "Hope for the best while preparing for the worst." At the end of a family meeting, the PA should share any change in plans with key clinical personnel and document decisions in the medical record.[8–10]

MANAGING NONPAIN SYMPTOMS AT THE END OF LIFE
Dyspnea

Dyspnea is a subjective sensation of breathlessness that differs from patient to patient, often accompanied by anxiety. This sensation arises from both central and peripheral chemoreceptors in response to an increase in $Paco_2$ or a decrease in either Pao_2 or pH. Some patients may experience dyspnea, however, when these parameters are normal, whereas other patients do not experience dyspnea even with severe blood gas abnormalities.[11]

In evaluating dyspnea, check for simple causes, such as the oxygen tubing not being connected, turned off, or kinked, as well as uncontrolled pain, constipation, or urinary retention. Further diagnostic work-up depends on a patient's goals and how close the patient is to death. In some cases, laboratory and imaging tests could diagnose an exacerbation of chronic obstructive pulmonary disease (COPD) or heart failure, pulmonary infection, or embolism. At the end of life, however, most treatment is symptomatic.[12]

Opioids relieve dyspnea by reducing the ventilatory response to both carbon dioxide and oxygen, by decreasing oxygen consumption, and by decreasing pulmonary vascular resistance.[13] The American College of Chest Physicians endorses opioids to treat dyspnea in selected patients with chronic heart or lung disease.[14] The benefit of opioids in relieving dyspnea is modest, however, unlike treating pain. In 1 study of patients with end-stage COPD, patients received either extended-release morphine (20 mg orally daily) followed by placebo. Morphine provided an improvement of 6.5 mm on a 0 mm to 100 mm visual analog scale of dyspnea compared with placebo.[15] It is best to start low, with 5 mg of oral morphine every 2 hours to 3 hours as needed, converting to a long-acting preparation if needed.

Sedating drugs are sometimes added to morphine. Dyspnea often coexists with anxiety in patients with terminal disease. The clinician should first use an opioid in these patients, but if the response to morphine is inadequate, a benzodiazepine, such as lorazepam or an antidepressant (tricyclic antidepressants or selective serotonin reuptake inhibitors) can be added. Benzodiazepines by themselves do not improve dyspnea, but there is a modest benefit when a benzodiazepine is added to an opioid.[16] The combination of opioids and benzodiazepines may increase mortality, but this risk may be acceptable to patients at the end of life.

Steroids may help selected patients. Dexamethasone or a similar glucocorticoid should be considered for dyspnea caused by asthma, superior vena cava syndrome, radiation pneumonitis, or carcinomatous lymphangitis.[12]

Oxygen is often administered to relieve dyspnea, with surprisingly little evidence of effectiveness. In a classic study, nonhypoxemic terminally ill patients with refractory dyspnea were randomized to receive either oxygen or room air. Dyspnea improved to the same degree with either treatment.[17] Another study compared the benefits of oxygen with an opioid in relieving dyspnea in dying patients, both in those with hypoxemia and those without. The opioid was modestly effective in both groups, whereas oxygen provided no benefit in either group (not even when there was hypoxemia).[18] In a simple, nonblinded study, when patients blew air into their face with a handheld fan, dyspnea decreased by 29% compared with air blown at their legs.[19]

Cough

When mucociliary clearance is inadequate, cough is a reflex to clear the airways. Common causes of cough in patients at the end of life include angiotensin-converting enzyme inhibitors, pulmonary infections, asthma/COPD, lung cancer, pulmonary edema, reflux, and aspiration.[20] Treatment options include inhaled β_2-agonists for bronchospasm and steroids for cough caused by lymphangitic tumor spread. When no further disease-specific treatment is available, the goal becomes suppression of cough to enhance comfort. Antitussives include peripherally and centrally acting drugs. The only peripheral antitussive is benzonatate (100–200 mg twice daily). Central drugs include dextromethorphan (10–20 mg every 4–6 hours) and opioids. In most cases, benzonatate should be tried before prescribing an opioid.[21] Other palliative treatments for refractory cough include gabapentin, diazepam, and honey.[22–24]

Respiratory Secretions

Dying patients lose the ability to swallow effectively, lose cough reflexes, and have an increase in cholinergic muscarinic activity, which impairs the ability to clear secretions. Turbulent breathing through these secretions produces noisy breathing, which occurs in 10% to 90% of dying patients. These secretions do not generally bother a dying patient, but the family may interpret the symptom as choking, drowning, or strangling. The team should maintain a calm and competent approach to reduce anxiety, avoiding the term, *death rattle*.[25] A scale to score the severity of respiratory secretions has been developed for use in evaluating the benefit of treatment (**Table 2**).[26]

Table 2 Scale for rating noisy breathing due to respiratory secretions	
Score	**Audibility of Breathing**
0	Inaudible
1	Audible only very close to the patient
2	Clearly audible at the end of the bed in a quiet room
3	Clearly audible at 20 ft (at the door) in a quiet room

Data from Back IN, Jenkins K, Blower A, et al. A study comparing hyoscine hydrobromide and glycopyrrolate in the treatment of death rattle. Palliat Med 2001;15:329–36.

Nonpharmacologic therapy

The patient may be positioned to 1 side or to semiprone to facilitate postural drainage. In the last few days of life, an option is to discontinue routine turning every 1 hour to 2 hours. If 1 position creates fewer secretions, that position should be preferred. Reducing or stopping artificial hydration may reduce excess secretions, especially among patients who have intravenous (IV) fluids for several days and have hypoalbuminemia. Aspiration of secretions with a suction catheter can clear the oropharynx, but this is usually avoided because it is noisy and uncomfortable.[25]

Pharmacologic therapy

Anticholinergic drugs block secretions by inhibiting the parasympathetic nervous system (**Table 3**). Glycopyrrolate does not cross the blood-brain barrier and has minimal central anticholinergic side effects, such as delirium.[27] Other anticholinergic agents cross the blood-brain barrier and have more potential to impair cognition. For unconscious patients, however, they are often used to quiet noisy breathing. Atropine drops can be administered sublingually. Scopolamine patches take 24 hours for serum levels to reach steady state.[27]

Adverse effects of anticholinergic drugs include dry mouth, urinary retention, photophobia, tachycardia, and constipation and, for those that cross the blood-brain barrier, headache, drowsiness, weakness, dizziness, and delirium. Although these drugs may reduce the production of new secretions, they cannot remove secretions already present.

Despite their widespread use, limited research has compared the effectiveness of anticholinergic medications. In 1 study, terminally ill patients with noisy secretions were randomized to atropine, scopolamine, or hyoscine butylbromide, without a placebo. All 3 drugs reduced the secretion score to low levels or zero by 24 hours in 70% of patients. Without a placebo, however, it is possible much of the effect simply reflected the possibility that noisy secretions spontaneously decrease.[28]

A recent study randomized hospice patients with noisy breathing to receive 2 drops of 1% sublingual atropine solution or placebo, with the primary outcome reduction in secretions at 4 hours. This outcome was reached at the same rate in each group.[29] Given limited benefit plus numerous side effects, anticholinergic drugs should not

Table 3
Drugs used to prevent or treat noisy secretions at the end of life

Drug	Brand Name	Route	Usual Starting Dose	Comments
Atropine		PO, SL	0.2 mg every 4–6 h 1% eye drops: 1–2 drops Every 4–6 h	Onset in 30 min
		SC, IV	0.1–0.5 mg every 4–6 h	Onset in 1 min
Glycopyrrolate	Robinul	PO	1 mg every 6 h	Onset in 30 min, maximum dose 8 mg/24 h
		SC, IV	0.2–0.4 mg every 4–6 h	Onset in 1 min
Hyoscyamine	Levsin	PO, SL	0.125 mg every 4–6 h	Onset in 30 min, maximum dose 1 mg/24 h
Scopolamine (hyoscine hydrobromide)	Transderm Scop	patch	1.5 mg patch changed every third day	Onset in 24 h, steady state takes several days
		SC, IV	0.25–0.4 mg every 4–6 h	Quicker onset

Abbreviations: PO, oral; SC, subcutaneous; SL, sublingual.

be routinely used in preventing or treating noisy respiratory secretions. Nonpharmacologic approaches should be the mainstay of treatment.

Nausea and Vomiting

Nausea and vomiting occur in more than 40% of cancer patients in the last few weeks of life and among 70% of all patients in palliative units. There is a discrete brainstem vomiting center that receives input from at least 4 pathways: the chemoreceptor trigger zone (CTZ), which samples the serum and cerebrospinal fluid for toxins; the vestibular system, which detects motion; the gastrointestinal (GI) tract, which senses stretch, local injury, and toxins; and the cortex, influenced by sensory input, anxiety, and increased intracranial pressure. Chemotherapy causes nausea mainly through the CTZ, with dopamine (D_2) as its receptor; a strong D_2-blocker, such as haloperidol, is often effective. On the other hand, GI obstruction or stasis causes nausea through activation of serotonin receptors; this kind of nausea responds better to a serotonin antagonist, such as ondansetron.[30]

Specific causes of nausea are often suggested by history. Persistent nausea worsened by the sight or smell of food and not relieved by vomiting suggests that the CTZ may be activated by emesis-inducing substances in the blood. Intermittent nausea associated with abdominal cramping and relieved by vomiting suggests bowel obstruction. Early morning nausea, vomiting, and headache suggest increased intracranial pressure. Nausea aggravated by motion suggests a vestibular origin, and nausea associated with anxiety suggests a brain lesion.[30]

Nonpharmacologic therapy

Nondrug approaches include avoiding strong smells or other environmental triggers and eating small, frequent cold foods in a pleasant, comfortable environment. For patients receiving chemotherapy, relaxation therapy, guided imagery, acupuncture, and acupressure may help.[30]

Pharmacologic therapy

If the etiology of a patient's nausea and vomiting is known and easily treatable, that treatment can be provided. It is appropriate to prescribe a drug (**Table 4**) around-the-clock for 24 hours to 48 hours, not just as needed, before concluding that it is ineffective.[30,31] A serotonin antagonist, such as ondansetron, is effective in chemotherapy-associated and radiation-associated nausea and vomiting. These drugs have a high therapeutic

Table 4
Choice of medications for nausea and vomiting, based on etiology

Etiology	Suggested Medications
Bowel obstruction	Metoclopramide, if incomplete; otherwise haloperidol, olanzapine, dexamethasone, octreotide
Brain tumor	Dexamethasone
Chemotherapy-induced	Ondansetron, dexamethasone, aprepitant
Impaired GI motility	Metoclopramide
Motion-associated	Scopolamine, diphenhydramine, promethazine
Opioids	Haloperidol, metoclopramide, prochlorperazine, olanzapine
Radiation associated	Ondansetron

Data from Wood GJ, Shega JW, Lynch B, et al. Management of intractable nausea and vomiting in patients at the end of life. "I was feeling nauseous all the time...nothing was working." JAMA 2007;298(10):1196–207.

index, with few adverse effects. Ginger at a dose of 0.5 g to 1.5 g per dose has evidence of effectiveness for acute chemotherapy-induced nausea.[32] For nausea caused by intracranial hypertension, dexamethasone may help.[30]

Aprepitant works by antagonizing the neurokinin-1 receptor. These expensive drugs are effective for chemotherapy-associated nausea, but they have not been studied widely for other uses in palliative care.[32]

Opioid-induced nausea is often transient, most common when opioids are initiated or the dose is increasing. One approach is to either reduce the opioid dose or switching to another opioid. Codeine and morphine may produce more nausea than others. For persistent opioid-induced nausea, the clinician may prescribe a strong D_2-blocker, such as haloperidol.[33]

Patients with malignant bowel obstruction often experience nausea and vomiting. For patients who are not undergoing surgery or stent placement, medical management includes an opioid, glycopyrrolate, octreotide, steroids, and/or haloperidol. Metoclopramide can replace haloperidol the obstruction is incomplete.[34]

If the etiology of nausea and vomiting is unclear, the first drug should be a D_2-antagonist, such as haloperidol, although some experts prefer prochlorperazine or metoclopramide. Using haloperidol for nausea is effective and widely acknowledged in the palliative care literature,[35] but its use may be resisted by staff in long-term care settings, where it is often avoided due to adverse effects. Topical haloperidol was found ineffective in a recent study.[36] The atypical neuroleptic olanzapine is an effective alternative to haloperidol.[37]

Constipation

Constipation is the passage of small, hard feces infrequently and/or with difficulty. The prevalence of constipation in palliative-care populations ranges from 30% to 90%.[38] Patients may be asked what they consider a normal bowel pattern as well as when constipation began. The most important part of the evaluation is a rectal examination to detect fecal impaction. An abdominal examination may detect an abdominal mass or evidence of bowel obstruction. A plain abdominal film can assess the severity of constipation.

Medical conditions can cause constipation. These include electrolyte disorders and conditions causing patients to withhold stool because of pain from anal fissures, hemorrhoids, and rectal prolapse. The extent of any work-up, including laboratory tests or procedures, such as colonoscopy, should be based on a patient's goals of care.

The most easily reversed cause of constipation in a palliative care patient is a medication side effect. Although constipation is a nearly universal adverse effect of opioids, many other constipation-causing medications can often be tapered or discontinued. Such medications include aluminum-containing or calcium-containing antacids, anticholinergics, antihistamines, antidepressants and antipsychotics, calcium channel blockers, clonidine, corticosteroids, diuretics, iron, levodopa, nonsteroidal anti-inflammatory drugs, ondansetron, and sympathomimetics.[39,40]

If impaction is detected on rectal examination, the clinician should perform digital disimpaction.[11] If the rectum is filled with hard stool, disimpaction should be followed by a saline enema, then by glycerin or bisacodyl suppositories, followed by oral senna. If the rectum is filled with soft stool, disimpaction is followed by oral senna, without an enema. If there is no fecal impaction, prescribe senna plus a nonabsorbable osmotic laxative is often effective.[41]

Nonpharmacologic therapy

Patients may be encouraged to attempt a bowel movement when peristalsis is most active—on awakening in the morning and after meals. Increasing fiber intake, although recommended for general treatment of constipation, is usually not a good idea for palliative patients. If fluid intake does not increase along with increased fiber intake, the fiber may harden stool. Although immobility and low levels of physical activity are associated with constipation, there is little evidence that exercise relieves constipation, and exercise is usually impractical for dying patients.[42]

Pharmacologic therapy

Laxatives work either by stimulating persistalsis or by softening stool. Stimulant laxatives include senna and bisacodyl. They increase intestinal motility and secretion of water into the bowel. Senna is the first choice, especially for those on opioids, starting with one 8.6-mg tablet at bedtime (2 tablets if a patient is taking opioids) and working up to as many as 2 tablets to 4 tablets 3 times per day. Stimulant laxatives should not be used in patients with bowel obstruction.[43]

Although senna and bisacodyl are the preferred laxatives in palliative care, other agents are available. Bulk laxatives, which contain either soluble fiber (psyllium, pectin, or guar) or insoluble fiber (cellulose) are hydrophilic, increasing stool water mass and enhancing intraluminal transit. Because these agents require substantial liquid intake, however, they are not appropriate for palliative patients.

Stool softeners, such as docusate, work by reducing surface tension. They have limited effectiveness, particularly for patients who have opioid-induced constipation. A recent trial showed that for patients on opioids, oral docusate added no further benefit to senna.[44]

Osmotic laxatives are hyperosmolar agents that work by drawing fluid into the bowel. They include nonabsorbable sugar-containing laxatives, such as sorbitol, lactulose, and polyethylene glycol 3350. If senna is ineffective for treating constipation in palliative care, one of these agents is the next step (sorbitol 30 mL orally daily). Other osmotic laxatives, such as magnesium hydroxide, magnesium citrate, and sodium bisphosphate, should be avoided because they cause electrolyte disturbances and diarrhea.[45]

Opioid-associated constipation

Patients prescribed opioids should receive prophylactic senna. If constipation persists, the next step is to increase the dose of senna or add an osmotic laxative. If these are ineffective, a peripheral opioid antagonist, such as methylnaltrexone, may be effective. This drug antagonizes peripheral μ-opioid receptors in the bowel, reversing the opioid side effect of constipation, but they do not cross the blood-brain barrier, leaving analgesia unaffected. A typical dose of methylnaltrexone (Relistor) is 8 mg subcutaneously as a single dose for patients weighing 38 kg to 62 kg, or 12 mg subcutaneously for patients weighing 62 kg to 114 kg.[46]

ARTIFICIAL NUTRITION AND HYDRATION

Like cardiopulmonary resuscitation and mechanical ventilation, artificial nutrition and hydration (ANH) is a medical treatment that patients may accept or refuse. An older adult may specify his preference in a living will, but the decision to use ANH is usually made by family members. ANH may be provided IV, either as standard fluids or total parenteral nutrition (TPN), or it may be provided through a nasogastric tube or percutaneous endoscopic gastrostomy (PEG) tube.

ANH is beneficial for many conditions, such as the acute phase of stroke or head injury, in critically ill patients with potentially treatable conditions, and in selected patients with advanced malignancy who are undergoing intensive radiation therapy or have proximal bowel obstruction. There is also a role for ANH in patients with amyotrophic lateral sclerosis (ALS) who are unable to eat and drink.[47,48]

The pathophysiology of anorexia and cachexia in patients with advanced disease is complex and poorly understood. Numerous cytokines. such as tumor necrosis factor α, interleukin (IL)-1, IL-6, and interferon-γ, are produced by both the patient and by cancer cells. This creates an ongoing inflammatory catabolic state, in which energy is being broken down rather than stored. Providing extra energy in this state is ineffective. This may be explained as, "Your father isn't dying because he isn't eating; he's not eating because he is dying."[49]

There is strong evidence that TPN is either ineffective or harmful in most patients with cancer. A review of 26 randomized trials of TPN provided to cancer patients undergoing chemotherapy demonstrated more infections and poorer tumor response in the TPN group. A review of more than 40 randomized trials of perioperative TPN in patients undergoing cancer surgery demonstrated no benefit in morbidity or mortality, with 1 exception: preoperative TPN in patients with upper GI cancers. A review of 15 trials of enteral perioperative nutritional support for cancer surgery benefits showed no benefits.[50]

ARTIFICIAL NUTRITION AND HYDRATION IN PATIENTS WITH DEMENTIA

Patients with advanced dementia resist or become indifferent to food, become unable to chew and swallow, and aspirate. Patients with dementia, however, who cannot feed themselves may live several years, particularly if they have dedicated caregivers and do not have other terminal illness. Inevitably, dementia progresses to the point that a patient does not take any oral feedings. There are 2 main options: keep trying to feed by mouth or initiate tube feedings.[47]

Family members are often concerned that their loved one is "starving to death," but evidence suggests that patients with end-stage dementia rarely experience hunger or thirst. Based on strong evidence, PAs should confidently recommend against feeding tubes for patients with end-stage dementia (**Box 3**). Tube feeding in these patients is associated with multiple risks and no clear benefits. Aspiration and pneumonia are more common with tube feeding compared with careful hand feeding, probably because there are more pharyngeal secretions and more gastroesophageal reflux in tube-fed patients.

A cohort study of more than 36,000 nursing home patients with advanced dementia that controlled for confounding variables found that PEG feeding did not improve

---

Box 3
The arguments against artificial nutrition in patients with advanced dementia

Feeding tubes in patients suffering from advanced dementia
• Increase morbidity, mortality, and hospitalization
• Cause discomfort because of the need for tube replacement or repositioning
• Do not improve quality of life or nutritional parameters
• Do not reduce the risk of aspiration of pneumonia
• Do not improve survival

Tube feeding in these patients causes harm and suffering by
• Causing social isolation by reducing the need for patients to participate in mealtime
• Causing the clear majority to require chemical or physical restraints
• Increasing the risk of a new pressure ulcer or worsening of an established ulcer
• Caregivers believing that end-of-life care was of poorer quality

Adapted from Merel SE, DeMers S, Vig E. Palliative care in advanced dementia. Clin Geriatr Med 2014;30(3):469–92; with permission.

survival. Early placement of the PEG (vs placement later in the disease) also made no difference in survival.[51] Pressure sores are neither prevented nor treated by PEG in patients with advanced dementia. A cohort study demonstrated that PEG feeding increased the number of new pressure sores and worsened healing among established pressure sores in patients with advanced dementia.[52] The PA should clarify that dementia is a fatal illness and that feeding problems indicate the disease has reached end-stage. One can reassure family members that not using a feeding tube will not cause suffering.

For patients still able to consume some oral feedings, interventions can make oral feeding easier and more comfortable. These include addressing yeast stomatitis, ill-fitting dentures, or medications causing dry mouth. Nonessential medications, such as bisphosphonates, statins, and anticoagulants. Finger foods, preferred foods, strong flavors, or foods with high caloric density, like ice cream may help. Using smaller bolus size, giving liquids if a patient prefers them, altering food texture, and providing personal assistance are other options.[53,54]

From a legal or ethical perspective, withholding ANH and withdrawing ANH are equivalent, but practically it is easier to not begin ANH than to withdraw it. There are times, however, when clinicians care for patients with advanced dementia already receiving ANH. The only predictable consequence of fluid restriction at the end of life is dry mouth, which can be managed by moistening the lips. A randomized trial of fluids versus no fluids in patients with advanced cancer (not patients with dementia) found no benefits in terms of improved symptoms, quality of life, or survival.[55] Some families may resist plans to discontinue feeding or fluids, but they may agree to reduce the infusion rate.

REFERENCES

1. Kapo J, Morrison LJ, Liao S. Palliative care for the older adult. J Palliat Med 2007; 10(1):185–209.
2. Reuben DB. Medical care for the final years of life. "When you're 83, it's not going to be 20 years. JAMA 2009;302(24):2686–94.
3. Kelley AS, Morrison RS. Palliative care for the seriously ill. N Engl J Med 2015; 373:747–55.
4. National Palliative Care Registry. Annual survey summary: results of the 2016 National Palliative Care Registry Survey. Available at: https://registry.capc.org/wp-content/uploads/2017/02/Growth-of-Palliative-Care-in-U.S.-Hospitals - 2016-Snapshot.pdf. Accessed February 1, 2018.
5. Teno JM, Connor SR. Referring a patient and family to high-quality palliative care at the close of life: "we met a new personality…with this level of compassion and empathy". JAMA 2009;301:651–9.
6. Center for Medicare and Medicaid Services. Medicare benefit policy manual chapter 9-coverage of hospice services under hospital insurance. Rev 2015; 209:05–8. Available at: https://www.cms.gov/Regulations-and-Guidance/Guidance/Manuals/downloads/bp102c09.pdf.
7. National Hospice and Palliative Care Organization. 2017 NHPCO facts and figures. Hospice in America. Available at: http://www.nhpco.org/sites/default/files/public/Statistics_Research/2016_Facts_Figures.pdf. Accessed February 1, 2018.
8. Billings JA. The end-of-life family meeting in intensive care part I: indications, outcomes, and family needs. J Palliat Med 2011;14(9):1042–50.
9. Billings JA. The end-of-life family meeting in intensive care part II: family-centered decision making. J Palliat Med 2011;14(9):1051–7.

10. Billings JA, Block SD. The end-of-life family meeting in intensive care part III: a guide for structured discussions. J Palliat Med 2011;14(9):1058–64.

11. Kamal AH, Maguire JM, Wheeler JL, et al. Dyspnea review for the palliative professional: assessment, burdens, and etiologies. J Palliat Med 2011;14(10): 1167–72.

12. Kamal AH, Maguire JM, Wheeler JL, et al. Dyspnea review for the palliative professional: treatment goals and therapeutic options. J Palliat Med 2012;15(1): 106–14.

13. Eckström MP, Bornefalk-Hermansson A, Abernethy AP, et al. Safety of benzodiazepines and opioids in very severe respiratory disease: a national prospective study. BMJ 2014;348:g445.

14. Mahler DA, Selecky PA, Harrod CG, et al. American College of Chest Physicians consensus statement on the management of dyspnea in patients with advanced lung or heart disease. Chest 2010;137(3):674–91.

15. Abernethy AP, Currow DC, Frith P, et al. Randomised, double blind, placebo controlled crossover trial of sustained release morphine for the management of refractory dyspnoea. BMJ 2003;327(7414):523–8.

16. Periyakoil VS, Skultety K, Sheikh J. Panic, anxiety, and chronic dyspnea. J Palliat Med 2005;8(2):453–9.

17. Abernethy AP, McDonald CF, Frith PA, et al. Effect of palliative oxygen versus room air in relief of breathlessness in patients with refractory dyspnea: a double-blind, randomised controlled trial. Lancet 2010;376:784–93.

18. Clemens KE, Quednau I, Klaschik E. Use of oxygen and opioids in the palliation of dyspnoea in hypoxic and non-hypoxic palliative care patients: a prospective study. Support Care Cancer 2009;17(4):367–77.

19. Galbraith S, Fagan P, Perkins P, et al. Does the use of a handheld fan improve chronic dyspnea? A randomized, controlled, crossover trial. J Pain Symptom Manage 2010;39(5):831–8.

20. Irwin RS, Baumann MH, Boulet L-P, et al. Diagnosis and management of cough executive summary. ACCP evidence-based clinical practice guidelines. Chest 2006;129(1 Suppl):1S–23S.

21. Estfan B, LeGrand S. Management of cough in advanced cancer. J Support Oncol 2004;2:523–7.

22. Ryan NM, Birring SS, Gibson PG. Gabapentin for refractory chronic cough: a randomised, double-blind, placebo-controlled trial. Lancet 2012;380:1583–9.

23. Estfan B, Walsh D. The cough from hell: diazepam for intractable cough in a patient with renal cell carcinoma. J Pain Symptom Manage 2008;36(5):553–8.

24. Paul IM, Beiler J, McMonagle A, et al. Effect of honey, dextromethorphan, and no treatment in nocturnal cough and sleep quality for coughing children and their parents. Arch Pediatr Adolesc Med 2007;161(12):1140–6.

25. Lokker ME, van Zuylen L, van der Rijt CC, et al. Prevalence, impact, and treatment of death rattle: a systematic review. J Pain Symptom Manage 2014;47(1): 105–22.

26. Back IN, Jenkins K, Blower A, et al. A study comparing hyoscine hydrobromide and glycopyrrolate in the treatment of death rattle. Palliat Med 2001;15:329–36.

27. Prommer E. Anticholinergics in palliative medicine: an update. Am J Hosp Palliat Med 2012;30(5):490–8.

28. Wildiers H, Dhaenekint C, Demeuleneare P, et al. Atropine, hyoscine butylbromide, or scopolamine are equally effective for the treatment of death rattle in terminal care. J Pain Symptom Manage 2009;38(1):124–33.

29. Heisler M, Hamilton G, Abbott A, et al. Randomized double-blind trial of sublingual atropine vs. placebo for the management of death rattle. J Pain Symptom Manage 2013;45(1):14–22.

30. Wood GJ, Shega JW, Lynch B, et al. Management of intractable nausea and vomiting in patients at the end of life. "I was feeling nauseous all the time...nothing was working." JAMA 2007;298(10):1196–207.

31. Gupta M, Davis M, LeGrand S, et al. Nausea and vomiting in advanced cancer: the Cleveland Clinic protocol. J Supp Oncol 2007;298(10):1196–207.

32. Jordan K, Janh F, Aapro M. Recent developments in the prevention of chemotherapy-induced nausea and vomiting (CINV): a comprehensive review. Ann Oncol 2015;26(6):1081–90.

33. Davis MP, Hallerberg G, Palliative Medicine Study Group of the Multinational Association of Supportive Care in Cancer. A systematic review of the treatment of nausea and/or vomiting in cancer unrelated to chemotherapy or radiation. J Pain Symptom Manage 2010;39(4):756–67.

34. Laval G, Arvieux C, Stefani L, et al. Protocol for the treatment of malignant inoperable bowel obstruction: a prospective study of 80 cases at Grenoble University Hospital Center. J Pain Symptom Manage 2006;31(6):502–12.

35. Vella-Brincat J, Macleod AD. Haloperidol in palliative care. Palliat Med 2004; 18(3):195–201.

36. Smith TJ, Ritter JK, Poklis JL, et al. ABH gel is not absorbed from the skin of normal volunteers. J Pain Symptom Manage 2012;43(5):961–6.

37. McKintosh D. Olanzapine in the management of difficult to control nausea and vomiting in a palliative care population: a case series. J Palliat Med 2016;19(1): 87–90.

38. Erichsén E, Milberg A, Jarrsma T, et al. Constipation in specialized palliative care: prevalence, definition, and patient-perceived symptom distress. J Palliat Med 2015;18(7):585–92.

39. Sykes NP. The pathogenesis of constipation. Support Oncol 2006;4(5):213–8.

40. Tamayo AC, Diaz-Zuluaga PA. Management of opioid-induced bowel dysfunction in cancer patients. Support Care Cancer 2004;12(9):613–8.

41. Larkin PJ, Sykes NP, Centeno C, et al. The management of constipation in palliative care: clinical practice recommendations. Palliat Med 2008;22(7):796–807.

42. Librach SL, Bouvette M, De Angelis C, et al. Consensus recommendations for the management of constipation in patients with advanced, progressive illness. J Pain Symptom Manage 2010;40(5):761–73.

43. Twycross R, Sykes N, Mihalyo M, et al. Stimulant laxatives and opioid-induced constipation. J Pain Symptom Manage 2012;43(2):306–13.

44. Tarumi Y, Wilson MP, Szafran O, et al. Randomized, double-blind, placebo-controlled trial of oral docusate in the management of constipation in hospice patients. J Pain Symptom Manage 2013;45(1):2–13.

45. Xing JH, Soffer EE. Adverse effects of laxatives. Dis Colon Rectum 2001;44: 1201–9.

46. Thomas J, Karver S, Cooney GA, et al. Methylnaltrexone for opioid-induced constipation in advanced illness. N Engl J Med 2008;358:2332–43.

47. Casarett D, Kapo J, Caplan A. Appropriate use of artificial nutrition and hydration – fundamental principles and recommendations. N Engl J Med 2005;353(24): 2607–12.

48. Assenat E, Thezenas S, Flori N, et al. Prophylactic percutaneous endoscopic gastrostomy in patients with advanced head and neck tumors treated by combined chemoradiotherapy. J Pain Symptom Manage 2011;42(4):548–56.

49. Suzuki H, Asakawa A, Amitani H, et al. Cancer cachexia – pathophysiology and management. J Gastroenterol 2013;48:579–84.
50. Koretz RL. Should patients with cancer be offered nutritional support: does the benefit outweigh the burden? J Gastroenterol Hepatol 2007;19:379–82.
51. Teno JM, Gozalo PL, Mitchell SL, et al. Does feeding tube insertion and its timing improve survival? J Am Geriatr Soc 2012;60(10):1918–21.
52. Teno MJ, Gozalo P, Mitchell SL, et al. Feeding tubes and the prevention or healing of pressure ulcers. Arch Intern Med 2012;172(9):697–701.
53. Palacek EJ, Teno JM, Casarett DJ, et al. Comfort feeding only: a proposal to bring clarity to decision-making regarding difficulty with eating for persons with advanced dementia. J Am Geriatr Soc 2010;58(3):580–4.
54. American Geriatrics Society Ethics Committee and Clinical Practice and Models of Care Committee. American Geriatrics Society feeding tubes in advanced dementia practice statements. J Am Geriatr Soc 2014;62(8):1590–3.
55. Bruera E, Hui D, Dalal S, et al. Parenteral hydration in patients with advanced cancer: a double-blind, placebo-controlled randomized trial. J Clin Oncol 2012; 31(1):111–8.

Functional Assessment and Pain Management

Lisa Cocco, MMS, PA-C*

KEYWORDS

- Pain management • Geriatric • Functional disability

KEY POINTS

- Many geriatric adults live independently despite a disability.
- Symptoms of pain and/or signs of functional decline can track the progression of the disability. Consider coadministering screening examinations with the Medicare Wellness Visits, and at the indication of pain, functional decline, or disability.
- Prepare yourself: Focus self-education on familiarizing yourself with existing, validated tools. Build a network of the local medical and complementary care providers.
- Prepare the clinic: Improve office flow by delegating tasks.
- Office delivery: Consider using the Centers of Disease Control and Prevention's Opioid Checklist to guide the conversation through the predictable areas of pain management. Anticipate establishing a plan to treat pain. Volunteer pain control management education before the patient feels desperate for relief. Follow-up, flexible goals, and coaccountability are paramount.

INTRODUCTION

Discussions and clinical pearls regarding the geriatric adult are often focused on the complex care of the *frail* adult, formally defined as a person in a state of physiologic decline and intolerance to medical interventions.[1] However, most geriatric patients live in a gray area between robust health and frailty, with a varied spectrum of disabilities and causes of chronic pain.

To demonstrate the incidence of disability versus frailty, a 2015 study by the Centers of Disease Control and Prevention (CDC) reported that 59.8% of geriatric adults were suffering from at least one "basic action disability or complex action limitation."[2] This figure represents more than 26.5 million American geriatric adults. However, a deeper look at the numbers reveals that only a small percentage of these adults required personal care assistance from another person (3.4% at ages 65–74, and 12.0% at ages

Disclosures: Author has no disclosures or conflicts of interest.
Pain Management, Internal Medicine
* 1998 Market Street, San Francisco, CA 94102.
E-mail address: lisa.r.cocco@gmail.com

Physician Assist Clin 3 (2018) 521–529
https://doi.org/10.1016/j.cpha.2018.05.006
2405-7991/18/© 2018 Elsevier Inc. All rights reserved.

75 and over).[2] Thus, a large percentage of the geriatric population is maintaining independence *despite* a disability.

With a rapidly growing geriatric population, providers must be aware of those that suffer in silence, and start to anticipate the need to track signs and symptoms of disability. To do so, there are 2 additional features that copresent with disability, namely "chronic pain" and "functional decline." In essence, only the patient can perceive the cumulative effect of disability; functional decline is the objective measure of disability, and chronic pain is a mental or physical manifestation that can forecast the trajectory of the disability. For clarity, key terms and concepts within this article are listed as follows:

- Disability: an acquired condition that is restricting the patient's ability to interact with his or her environment.
- Functional Capacity: documented by a provider, this is an objective measurement of the ability to perform physical and cognitive tasks. Common measures of capacity can be surveyed by screening examinations (eg, activities of daily living, documentation of hobbies and social activities) or physical examinations (eg, the Get-Up-and-Go test).
- Chronic pain: a mental or physical sensation that is unpleasant, traditionally longer than 3 months. In this definition, chronic pain is a common manifestation of disability, reflecting disease severity from the subjective perception of the patient.

Arthritis is a prime example of a common, insidious physical disability that can manifest as a chronic pain syndrome and untreated demoralization. In 2016, nearly half (49.6%) of geriatric adults in the United States had been physician diagnosed with an arthritis-causing condition at some point in his or her life,[3] although there is little research or surveys to yet determine how well this disease and its comorbidities have been managed.

Geriatric-associated disabilities that do not usually activate physical pain nociceptors (blindness, deafness, severe Alzheimer dementia, and similar) can also carry a high-risk comorbidity of depression. Depression is another well-studied cause or trigger of both pain and functional limitation.[4] Therefore, the estimated incidence of chronic mental and emotional pain is very high in the geriatric population well before the individual is markedly debilitated or frail.

Disability can be considered a chronic condition, with a trajectory that can be affected by appropriate screening, follow-up, intervention, and anticipatory patient education. For the protection of both provider and patient, the primary care provider will need to use the existing resources efficiently to deliver fast and objective functional assessments to detect and reduce the forecasted burden of disability, particularly in the geriatric patients with mild levels of disability that remain functionally independent.

CONTENT

There are many excellent, independent risk stratification tools available in the literature to assess chronic pain, disability, and functional capacity in the geriatric adult. However, no screening or monitoring tool is effective without a means of interpreting the results and developing an appropriate treatment plan. A screening tool is also ineffective if the provider administers the examination at inappropriate intervals: either too quickly or too far apart. Administering screening examinations and transitioning treatments for the fluidity of chronic conditions is best addressed by establishing treatment guidelines.

At this time, no guidelines have been developed to address screening geriatric adults for signs and symptoms of mild disability. When considering pain as a symptom of disability, the Medicare listing of Current Quality Measures states a general pain screening is only required for the patient already using hospice services.[5] The American Academy of Pain recognizes the multifactorial burden of pain, but most of their guidelines are limited to the treatment of a single medical diagnosis, not screening examinations by age and functional capacity.[6] The American Academy of Family Physicians provides a format for a "Geriatric Assessment," which should be implemented "at the suspicion of a potential problem."[7] It is a lengthy, multidimensional assessment that includes assessment of activities of daily living, physical examination, quality-of-life assessment, and depression screening.[7] However, even this extensive examination is cumbersome to implement "at the suspicion of a problem" this exam requires its own office visit.

Despite the lack of guidelines and strong recommendations for nearly impractical exams, existing screening tools can be re-purposed for fill this need.

Confident execution of validated screening tools can prolong independence, forecast trajectory from functional to frailty, improve patient-provider relationships, and create an environment with a smoother transition to peaceful end-of-life care.

Establishing a Baseline: Add Pain Management Screening into the Medicare Wellness Visits

Providers can prepare themselves and their work environments by implementing the steps listed in later discussion as a complement to Medicare's chronic care management initiatives. Medicare services have already been incredibly thorough in disseminating medical management expectations to patients and providers. As a result, most patients are cooperative during these office visits. Offer patients at aged 65 the Initial Preventative Physical Examination (IPPE, also called the "Welcome of Medicare Visit"), and offer the oral Annual Wellness Visit 12 months thereafter. The Resources section provides the link to complete the checklist of requirements to successfully administer the IPPE[8] and the Annual Wellness Visit.[9] A simple checklist format can help reduce both the complexity and the duration of the visit. A similar format can also help address chronic pain and functional assessment as risk factors for disability. If documented correctly, providers will be compensated for additional preventative examinations performed during the Medicare screening examination.

Establishing a Baseline: Administering the Examination at First Sign of Concern

Providers can also consider implementing the steps below during any situation wherein the patient requests pain control; if there are signs to imply that pain may be present; or if functional capacity is reduced per examination or screening findings.

Common manifestations of pain in the geriatric adult may include the following:

- Walking with cane
- Walking with a limp
- Rubbing body during the interview of an examination
- Anger or short temper
- Comments of "aging pains," or reference to age when responding to open-ended questions regarding health
- Mentioning a recent death of family or friend
- Mentioning retirement without replacement of fulfilling hobby

Before the next office visit, review the suggestions below to improve provider and office preparation. Supplemental discussion will be guided by the text in italic font.

Self-Preparation

- How do you perceive the geriatric population? Do you feel confident to treat a geriatric adult with a moderate disability as aggressively as the patient can tolerate?
- *Are you willing to allow the patient equal responsibility and autonomy in their care, as one would for a younger adult?*
- Have you built your network of local medical providers, with whom you can discuss or refer complex cases?
- *Collect resources and educate yourself on local options for complementary care; call local providers to make their acquaintance and learn more about their philosophies.*
- Have you completed Drug Enforcement Agency training, as provided by that state or state-based representative group?
- Are you registered and able to access the patients' controlled substance use report?
- Do you feel confident with the variety of opioids and their role outside of the perioperative setting?
- *Collect all available print screening tools that you believe would pertain to your patient population and then modify accordingly.*

The Provider Should Have the Similar Cooperative Expectations of a Functional Geriatric Adult as of a Younger Adult

Respect the patient's preserved ability to comprehend medical advice and implement multiple means for self-improvement. The provider should not diminish the patient's symptoms to "just aging pains" nor too quickly resort to palliative care as if treating a frail adult. The patient-provider relationship is paramount, but it is important to remember that this is a clinical relationship, that trust is critical, but both parties should make written and demonstrative efforts to achieve the ultimate goal. This relationship requires the patient to hold accountability for their health, including the use and misuse of the medical resources provided at the office visit. Adhering to this philosophy will protect the providers against exhaustion and malpractice.

Collect and Print Available Screening Tools That You Believe Would Pertain to Your Patient Population and Then Modify Accordingly

Although use of a single screening tool is consistent and less cumbersome, providers should become familiar with the multiple screening tools available. Complete an Internet search for "Functional Improvement Questionnaire" or "Pain Assessment Tools" to determine which best suits your practice. Having foreknowledge of when to use these tools and appropriate interpretation will also guide the visit toward meaningful action.

Few of these tools allow the space to note the medications that were taken in conjunction with the intervention. Medications are a cornerstone of medicine and can be complementary or competing against the patient's ultimate disability. A bulleted summary of all active methods for symptom control should be listed on any screening examination that has been administered to the patient. It is more effective to document the specific combination of interventions that created the effect rather than only documenting the change between the office visits.

Collect Resources and Educate Yourself on Local Options for Complementary Care

Most independent, yet chronically disabled patients desire to maintain their independence and functional capacity for as long as possible. Patients are frightened to see themselves as "frail." They are further frightened that medications and surgery are the only recourse that their providers can recommend. Thus, many patients often present their concerns to their provider in 2 ways: (1) they will mitigate the severity of their pain or disability to completely avoid interventions, or (2) they will present their concerns in a dramatic, hyperbolic way in order to "qualify" for surgery or medication. Either way, the patient has been living with pain, is seeking treatment, and simply requires education on the variety of treatment options that are approved and recommended by the medical community.

The following options are all highly recommended as first-line therapies: social inclusion programs, local exercise programs and pools, aqua therapy, acupuncture, chiropractor, volunteering opportunities, local group counseling advocates. A great barrier to referral is lack of provider trust and knowledge in these services. Just as it is unfair to stereotype a patient, it is also unfair to stereotype a potentially excellent therapy for complementary care. Conduct an Internet search for these treatments near the clinic and be willing to call these providers to determine the services offered and which patients would benefit from their services. A simple phone call or e-mail to introduce yourself and your patient population is sufficient, and request the other provider to explain their philosophies to patient care. It is perfectly reasonable to decide against referring a patient to a particular facility, but it is imperative that the provider remains open minded and determines *for oneself* how to best use the resources and providers around her to optimize patient care.

Self-education will allow the provider to have meaningful conversations with the patient in what other medical providers are able to offer, and the patient will be more willing to discuss the therapies that they received from other providers.

Finally, it is also helpful to seek understanding of how insurance companies and Health Savings Accounts can be applied to mitigate any cost for complementary therapies. Be sure to print literature that is language appropriate for the patient and family.

Office Preparation

- Has the patient already completed their IPPE? If so, are they now eligible for the Annual Wellness Examination?
- *Discuss with your team how to delegate roles to improve office flow.*
- *Who will access the State Controlled Substance Reporting Program?*
- Do you have the opioid agreement available to present, review, and sign in the office?
- How will you document in the problem list that the patient is taking a controlled substance?
- Will the patient be able to complete a urine toxicology screen in your office?

Discuss with Your Team How to Delegate Roles to Improve Office Flow

Much of the burden of the screening examinations can be delegated to other team members to maximize provider time for assessment and counseling. After creating physical copies of the provider's preferred screening examinations and educational materials, discuss with the office staff and medical assistants how to deliver these surveys to the patient at check-in or in the room while waiting for the provider. Have compassion for the team members, appreciating that they, too, have multiple tasks to balance. If the provider is ever altering the work-flow of the office, the provider should discuss why the screening tools are used with the team. If the relationship is appropriate, the staff can be trained to recognize and initiate the appropriate screening tool. Full office buy-in will improve excitement and adherence to the screening tools.

Become Familiar with the State-Controlled Substance Reporting Program

The patient's profile should be checked against the State's Controlled Substances Reporting Database at least annually and then at random once in the year if the patient is prescribed any controlled substance. It is a helpful record of who is prescribing the type, potency, and frequency of a controlled medication.

The database is free and discrete to access, but it can be cumbersome for the provider. A way to mitigate the burden on providers is to request the medical team to access the report before the patient visit.

Providers should note the limitations of the reporting system, because some pharmacies or institutions may have not have reported or be exempt from reporting a scheduled medication that they dispensed. For example, narcotics filled by the Veteran's Association or hospital pharmacies are often not reported to the State database. There is also no means of interstate communication, and the provider can only view the controlled substances that were provided in the state in which he or she practices.

Office Delivery

- *Guide the visit with one standard checklist.*
- *Functional Improvement Questionnaire Follow-up:* Where are the gaps in treatment? Are there gaps in the questionnaire and is a new assessment is warranted?
- *If opioids are to be started, do not skip the controlled substances agreement form.*
- *The urinalysis is still important in the geriatric adult at baseline and at random intervals.*
- Have you either offered or encouraged the complementary care to improve quality of life? (See the "collect resources" bullet under "Self-preparation".) Dispense as literature for the patient to review at home and encourage the patient and family to articulate their preferred management techniques.
- *Seek consultation in case of doubt.*

Guide the Visit and Goals with One Standard Checklist

The CDC's Checklist for prescribing opioids for chronic pain[10] is a checklist tool developed from the CDC's 2015 guidelines for initiating and prescribing chronic opioids. Because of the strong push to avoid opioid use, this checklist is a concise reminder of multiple treatment modalities and patient/provider protections regarding pain management. The provider can adapt this checklist in the following manner:

1. Review the "Reference" Panel with the patient first and make a separate list of non-opioid interventions that have been tried and failed.
2. Consider the remaining panels as recommended alternatives to pain control to guide the conversation. Determine what the patient does and does not understand about pain control techniques. Do not hesitate to discuss all points on the checklist.

The checklist also allows the provider to discuss pain control with narcotics *before* (or in immediate response to) the patient's request. Most patients are familiar with narcotics due to surgical or dental procedures, or testimonials from friends and family. Furthermore, it is often their only known technique of pain control outside of over-the-counter medications. Many patients are hesitant to address opioids until they feel a sense of desperation, with resulting impatience and defensive frustration when the provider (also often frustrated) responds with an ad hoc discussion of anti-opioid sentiments. Without a confident format, an office visit of this nature can become lengthy and fatiguing well before a plan is developed. Thus, this checklist offers an excellent template for focused discussion, but is also a tactile demonstration that the provider is *taking action* on the patient's request.

Based on the results of the checklist, the provider and patient can agree on the initial step to manage pain to improve functionality. The form can be scanned into the chart, and the current plan for pain control documented and developed.

Functional Improvement Questionnaire Delivery Follow-up

Each new intervention or dose adjustment should be reassessed 1 to 4 weeks later with the provider's selected FIQ. Follow-up visits at this interval are recommended by the CDC, and can be cited in the office note for purposes of reimbursement.[10] (see Web site checklist as https://stacks.cdc.gov/view/cdc/38025). Again, remember to add the list of the patient's medications in a bulleted list as well as any life changes that may have affected the outcome of this scoring.

This form can be completed with the patient, or the capable patient can complete the form before the office visit. Review the steps above in coordinating with the clinic team members.

Now is the time to compare the outcome of the intervention against the goals established at previous visits.

If Opioids Are to Be Started, Complete the Controlled Substances Agreement Form

The controlled substances agreement form is a dedicated explanation of your concerns with any prescribed medication (opioids, marijuana [where legal], antineuropathic agents, and so forth), the indicated uses, and expectations. Expectations should include ideal duration of use; early refills and vacation refill procedures; who will dispense the medication, including the chosen pharmacy; as well as the maximum dose he or she is allowed to take for both unexpected flares (eg, thunderstorm pressure changes) and anticipatory flares (eg, taking grandchildren to theme park). The patient and provider should establish expectations of each other, including the following:

- The intermittent administration of objective assessments, such body fluid analysis
- The provider should state if there are any medications or interventions that he or she is unwilling to prescribe
- Finally, expectations should segue into the clinical and psychiatric goals for pain control: what is an acceptable level of pain? Is it realistic?

The patient should be reassured that the agreement is not a legally binding contract in any way. All providers and staff members should avoid the term "contract" and use the term "agreement."

Providers should first determine if their facility has already created a Controlled Substance Agreement form and dispense or adapt that form as required. Additional templates are available through online searches. Consider beginning the search with the American Academy of Pain Medicine's adaptable template.

The Urinalysis Is Still Important in the Geriatric Adult at Baseline and at Random Intervals

The primary concerns of the medication toxicology screen address the question, "Is the patient taking the medication(s) as discussed in the agreement form?" In general, annual urine toxicology screen, one at random, and also after a fall or traumatic event to determine that medication, either prescribed or "borrowed" from another source, was not a contributory factor to the incident. Remember to discuss the potential insurance coverage for laboratory testing.

A common concern for both patients and providers is the interpretation of aberrant results of a urine toxicology report. Providers must respect the patient's human dignity, personality, and willpower to choose how they take their medication. Providers must also respect their own moral compass and confidently articulate when continued prescribing of a medication is contrary to best medical practice for this patient. For example, a patient may sell it to bolster meager income, and the urine toxicology screen may show either no medication or few by-products. The patient has knowingly misused medication, and now the provider is aware, but the ethos of the circumstances was nonmalicious. This circumstance need not ruin the rapport with the patient. First begin the conversation by acknowledging the complexity of the situation and then produce and review to the controlled substance agreement form to which both you and the patient agreed. Briefly educate the patient regarding the harm of selling the medications and the endangerment of your medical license. Then defer back to the Checklist, consider the medication a failed technique, and continue with *other techniques*. As always, clearly establish the next steps with the patient and document the circumstances in the progress note, with a summary in an obvious area of the medical record (see techniques in later discussion).

Make the Plan a Permanent Part of the Medical Record

There are simple techniques that can alert other providers of the goals and exclusivity of the treatment regimen. Consider adding the diagnosis of "Chronic Pain," "Opioid Use," or "High-Risk Medication Use" to the Problem List. Under the diagnosis, add a note to clarify the dispensing information of the interventions/medications used to treat the pain, including the name of the prescriber and when the next refill is due. Avoid adding the information as a note under a specific condition (such as "arthritis") because there may be multiple comorbid conditions that the medication is "treating." Again, consider chronic pain as its own separate condition that requires treatment instead of associating it with a more precise pathologic condition.

To help keep the list of interventions that have been trialed and failed in easy access, consider adding this list to the "social history" and adding details as required.

Seek Consultation in Case of Doubt

The variety of patient pathologies, personalities, and expectations may still result in a tumultuous relationship. Referring the patient for consultation may offer reprieve for the general medicine provider. Such specialists can include geriatricians, pain management providers, pain psychiatrists, chiropractors, or integrative medicine specialists. With all referrals, open-mindedness and respect to the recommendations of the specialist will improve the provider's knowledge as well as the patient's coordination of care.

SUMMARY

The proper management of chronic pain in the mildly disabled geriatric adult addresses many dimensions of care, but it can fit within the confines of a short office visit *and* be executed without exhausting the provider. Self-education on local programs and complementary care will be essential in the provider's clinical opinions for treatment. Preexisting tools and preoffice preparation strategies will prepare both the office and the provider for both routine and spontaneous screening of disability, functional capacity, and pain in the geriatric adult. The patient ignorant to the flexibility of Western medicine may present with denial or exaggeration of pain, but will find security in the provider's focused screening checklist tool. The primary care provider is in an ideal position to influence the transition from the functionally disabled to the frail-disabled adult, and the author has provided some pearls of wisdom and tools that combine the worlds of pain management specialty and Internal Medicine. At all times, provider and patient should maintain a sense of direction and purpose and request specialist consultation as needed to avoid a stagnant plan or a damaged relationship.

REFERENCES

1. Clegg A, Young J, Iliffe S, et al. Frailty in elderly people. Lancet 2013;381:752. Available at: https://www.uptodate.com/contents/frailty/abstract/1?utdPopup=true.
2. Disability and functioning (noninstitutionalized adults aged 18 and over). Atlanta (GA): Center for Disease Control; 2017. Available at: https://www.cdc.gov/nchs/fastats/disability.htm. Accessed November 6, 2017.
3. Barbour KE, Helmick CG, Boring M, et al. Vital signs: prevalence of doctor-diagnosed arthritis and arthritis-attributable activity limitation — United States, 2013–2015. MMWR Morb Mortal Wkly Rep 2017;66:246–53. Available at: https://doi.org/10.15585/mmwr.mm6609e1.
4. Trivedi MH. The link between depression and physical symptoms. Prim Care Companion J Clin Psychiatry 2004;6(Suppl 1):12–6. Available at: https://www.ncbi.nlm.nih.gov/pmc/articles/PMC486942/.
5. Hospice quality reporting program, current measures. Atlanta (GA): Centers for Medicare and Medicare Services; 2018. Available at: https://www.cms.gov/Medicare/Quality-Initiatives-Patient-Assessment-Instruments/Hospice-Quality-Reporting/Current-Measures.html. Accessed January 20, 2018.
6. Clinical guidelines. American Academy of Pain Medicine. Available at: http://www.painmed.org/library/clinical-guidelines/. Accessed November 9, 2017.
7. Elsawy B, Higgins K. Geriatric assessment. Am Fam Physician 2011;83(1):48–56. Available at: http://www.aafp.org/afp/2011/0101/p48.html. Accessed October10, 2017.
8. The ABCs of the annual wellness visit. Medical Learning Network. Atlanta (GA): Centers for Medicare and Medicare Services; 2017. Available at: https://www.cms.gov/Outreach-and-Education/Medicare-Learning-Network-MLN/MLNProducts/downloads/AWV_chart_ICN905706.pdf. Accessed January 19, 2018.
9. The ABCs of the initial provider preventative exam. Medical Learning Network. Atlanta (GA): Centers for Medicare and Medicare Services; 2017. Available at: https://www.cms.gov/Outreach-and-Education/Medicare-Learning-Network-MLN/MLNProducts/Downloads/MPS_QRI_IPPE001a.pdf. Accessed January 19, 2018.
10. Checklist for prescribing chronic Opioids. Poster publicizing: Dowell D, Haegerich TM, Chou R. CDC guideline for prescribing opioids for chronic pain—United States, 2016. MMWR Recomm Rep 2016;65(No. RR-1):1–49. Available at: https://stacks.cdc.gov/view/cdc/38025. Accessed November 6, 2017.

Depression in Older Adults
A Treatable Medical Condition

David A. Casey, MD

KEYWORDS

- Depression • Antidepressants • Electroconvulsive therapy

KEY POINTS

- Depression is not a normal part of the aging process.
- Depression in older adults is a treatable medical condition; a variety of psychotherapeutic and psychotherapeutic options are available.
- Electroconvulsive therapy is a useful treatment.
- The older patient must be viewed in their medical, functional, and social context for effective management.
- Cognition must be assessed along with mood in the older depressed patient.

INTRODUCTION

Depression is one of the most significant causes of emotional suffering in late life and may also be a contributing factor to the morbidity of many medical disorders.[1] Depressed elders often experience markedly diminished function and quality of life as well as mood symptoms. Increased mortality from both suicide and medical illness is also an important concomitant of depressive disorders in late life. Depression in older adults may be more persistent than depression earlier in life, often running a chronic, remitting course.[2] Clinical depression is not a part of normal aging but should be considered a treatable medical illness, although it certainly may be associated with problems of aging, such as loss, grief, and physical illness. The significance of late life depression is heightened by the fact that there are an increasing number of elders in the United States and many other countries.[3,4] The information in this article is particularly relevant to frail, medically ill, or cognitively impaired elders as well as the "old-old." The "old-old" is a somewhat ill-defined group, but here is used for those patients in their 80s or older. The use of age 65 as the onset of old age in geriatric medicine and psychiatry is arbitrary. Many such patients who are otherwise well may not require the specialized approach of the geriatrician.

This article originally appeared in *Primary Care Clinics: Clinics in Office Practice*, Volume 44, Issue 3, September 2017.

Department of Psychiatry and Behavioral Sciences, Geriatric Psychiatry Program, University of Louisville School of Medicine, 401 East Chestnut Street, Suite 610, Louisville, KY 40202, USA
E-mail address: dacase01@exchange.louisville.edu

Physician Assist Clin 3 (2018) 531–542
https://doi.org/10.1016/j.cpha.2018.05.009
2405-7991/18/© 2018 Elsevier Inc. All rights reserved.

DIAGNOSTIC CONCEPTS

Major depression is the most significant form of depression recognized in the Diagnostic and Statistical Manual of Mental Disorders, 5th edition (DSM-5), the handbook of psychiatric diagnosis of the American Psychiatric Association used in the United States and elsewhere. DSM-5 defines major depression based on the presence of 5 or more core depressive symptoms during a 2-week period, including either depressed mood or loss of interest or pleasure, along with significant weight loss or gain (without dieting) or appetite change, insomnia or hypersomnia, psychomotor agitation or retardation, fatigue or loss of energy, feelings of worthlessness or inappropriate guilt, diminished ability to think or concentrate or indecisiveness, and recurrent thoughts of death or suicide.[5] No distinction is made in the DSM-5 depression criteria based on age or aging. One of the most significant and controversial changes in DSM-5 was the removal of the "bereavement exclusion." In DSM-IV and other earlier versions of the handbook, persons who had suffered a recent loss with grief reaction were excluded from the diagnosis of major depression. This change may affect older adults more than other groups.

In the past, some investigators regarded major depression as more common among the elderly than other groups. However, it now appears that the prevalence of major depression among those 65 years or older is approximately 1% to 4%, a prevalence similar to (or perhaps even lower than) other groups. However, some special groups of older adults have higher rates of depressive symptoms. Elders with chronic medical illnesses have rates of depression of about 25%, and nursing home residents have a prevalence of approximately 25% to 50%.[2,6–8]

"Minor depression" is another important concept in geriatric psychiatry. This condition is sometimes referred to as "subsyndromal or subthreshold depression." It is not a designated diagnostic category in DSM-5, but is denoted as a section under the category "other specified depressive disorders." It is usually described as having the presence of 1 of the 2 principal depressive symptoms plus 1 to 3 additional symptoms, although this definition is not universally accepted.[5] This condition appears to be common, although rates of minor depression differ widely in studies. Despite its name, minor depression is associated with levels of disability similar to that of major depression.[5,9,10]

Dysthymia (alternately known as persistent depressive disorder in DSM-5) is a chronic form of depression that is less severe than major depression and lasts 2 or more years.[5] Although it more commonly begins earlier in life, it may persist into old age.[11]

The overall prevalence of all clinically significant depressive symptoms among older adults has been estimated at 8% to 16%.[2] African American elders have been noted to have lower rates of depression and are less likely to take antidepressant medication.[12] Older women are more likely to be diagnosed with depression than are older men. Owing to this higher diagnosis rate as well as having a longer lifespan, most diagnosed elder depressives are women.

Age of onset is also an important concept in geriatric depression, with early and late life onset groups. Depressive disorders beginning earlier in life may be persistent or recurrent, continuing into old age. In early onset cases, depressive symptoms tend to be similar through the course of illness. Some new onset cases in late life may represent differences in cause, possibly based on brain aging or illness. An important example of late life onset illness is "vascular depression," thought to be related to cerebrovascular changes.[13,14] These patients seem to be more likely to have cognitive dysfunction (especially loss of executive function), along with reduced verbal fluency, psychomotor retardation, functional loss, and anhedonia. In addition, these patients seem to be less likely to have a family history of depression or psychotic symptoms.

Depression in late life often occurs in the context of multiple medical illnesses. Often, depressive symptoms are misattributed to the aging process itself or viewed as a normal response to loss or illness.[1] Older adult patients may also focus on the physical symptoms associated with a depressive illness, accompanied by minimization of the emotional aspects of the illness. The term "masked depression" has been used to describe this situation, although the use of this term has diminished owing to a lack of precision as a diagnostic concept.[15] Although stigma may have diminished somewhat over the past 2 decades, many elders still feel uncomfortable with any psychiatric label that they think stigmatizes them and may engage in self-stigmatization. Elderly patients who are clearly suffering from a depressive disorder may describe themselves as anxious or "feeling bad" rather than sad, a condition that has been referred to as "depression without sadness."[16] In the context of significant medical illness, depression may be overlooked. The DSM-5 approach to diagnosis by using specific criteria, which is designed to make diagnosis more objective, may occasionally become an obstacle in diagnosing older patients. The question of whether a particular symptom such as loss of energy or appetite "counts" toward the diagnosis of depression may be raised if a physical illness may potentially explain it. Geriatric psychiatrists commonly take the approach that a symptom should be counted if it is present, regardless of other possible explanations.[17]

The diagnosis of depression in older adults is also complicated by the presence of loss and grief. Obviously, such losses are a common part of aging, and grief following a major loss is normal.[1] However, the removal of the bereavement exclusion in DSM-5 was made because of the fact that loss or grief may trigger a clinically relevant depressive episode.

In addition to mood symptoms, older depressives may report preoccupation with bodily function (eg, constipation, pain, insomnia, or fatigue), multiple diffuse complaints, weight loss, anxiety, obsessional ruminations, difficulty making decisions, or marked negativity. Other symptoms may also include a preoccupation with finances, executive cognitive dysfunction, melancholia (lack of mood variation, social interactions, and psychomotor changes), and loss of function at a level similar to severe medical illness. Terms such as "failure to thrive" or "depletion syndrome" have sometimes been used to describe older depressed patients who have a combination of loss of appetite, weight loss, and marked apathy or loss of interest.[18,19] Elderly depressed patients as a group have much more significant functional loss than younger patients. Functional deficits may include such things as giving up activities, staying in bed, exaggerated helplessness, dependency, and extreme negativism. This loss of function with depression among older adults can be profound and disabling.

A depressive illness may sometimes be accompanied by delusions or hallucinations, a condition known as psychotic or delusional depression. Commonly, although not always, these psychotic symptoms have depressive themes. Illogical thinking may also occur. A syndrome known as catatonia may occasionally be associated with psychotic depression (in addition to other psychiatric or medical conditions such as bipolar disorder). Catatonia involves varying degrees of withdrawal and mutism, sometimes accompanied by rigidity. Rigidity may also be accompanied by a tendency to hold the limbs in unusual postures, particularly if placed there by an examiner (often described as waxy flexibility) or repeat or sustain illogical behaviors (stereotypy). Patients with psychotic depression may experience delusions of guilt, poverty, decay, or disease. Psychotic depression is common among depressed elderly inpatients, occurring in 20% to 45% of these patients. However, psychotic depression is much less common in outpatients. Treatment of psychotic depression may require a combination of an antipsychotic medication with an antidepressant. Electroconvulsive therapy (ECT) is thought to be the most effective therapy for this condition, especially if accompanied by catatonic symptoms.[20,21]

The role of genetics in late life depression is poorly understood. Although early life onset depression is often associated with a family history, this may not be the case with late life onset depression. No particular genetic risk factor in late life onset depression has been discovered.[22]

MEDICAL ILLNESS AND DEPRESSION

Medical illnesses commonly accompany depression in late life.[23] Stroke, diabetes, cancer, chronic lung disease, Alzheimer disease (AD), Parkinson disease, arthritis, and fractures are all associated with depressive symptoms or a depressive illness. Endocrine conditions such as hypothyroidism, aging-related changes in the adrenal axis, and reduced levels of testosterone may play a role in some cases. Weight loss is commonly associated with elder depression and may contribute to vulnerability to other medical conditions.[2,24,25] This interplay between depression and medical illness may be bidirectional. The interrelationship between ischemic heart disease and depression seems to be particularly important. Depression seems to contribute to the morbidity and mortality of certain cardiovascular conditions and may be a consequence of these illnesses as well.[26] However, it is not entirely clear that treatment with antidepressants will necessarily ameliorate these effects.[27] Some community studies show an association between depression in elders and overall mortality,[28] although associated factors such as smoking, chronic medical disease, and lack of social support may confound these observations. Depressed patients are also heavy consumers of medical care, and a disproportionate number of primary care visits for physical complaints are driven at least in part by depression.[29]

Many commonly prescribed medications used by elders may contribute to depressive symptoms. This list includes (among others) cancer/antineoplastic drugs, corticosteroids, antiparkinsonians, metoclopramide, interferon, and various cardiovascular and antihypertensive drugs. Of course, alcohol and other substances of abuse may contribute to depressive symptoms. A comprehensive review of the patient's medication list, including over-the-counter medications, is a necessary part of any evaluation of depression.[30] This review also considers factors of adherence. How the drug is actually taken (or not taken) is important to understand. Patients may take medicine originally prescribed for another person or for an earlier episode of illness. Factors of cost, accessibility, complexity of the regimen, and cognitive impairment may all impact adherence.

COGNITIVE SYMPTOMS AND DEPRESSION

Depression often has a negative impact on cognition, especially among older adults. Depression may even occasionally be misdiagnosed as a dementing illness. Some observers have suggested that depression with cognitive impairment may be a harbinger of incipient dementia (especially AD) as either a risk factor or an early indicator, even if the cognitive impairment improves as the depression is treated. Several recent studies lend credence to the view that depression, especially depression recurrent over a period of years, is associated with an increased risk of later developing dementia and AD.[31–33] The concept of "depressive pseudodementia,"[34] which was commonly used in the past, is no longer widely applied. It is now appreciated that the presence of both depressive and cognitive symptoms most commonly represents a mingling of disease processes rather than one illness masquerading as another. Frequently, depressive symptoms are observed in a person with an established diagnosis of dementia. The term "depression of Alzheimer's disease (AD)" has been proposed for patients who meet the diagnostic criteria for AD and also have at least 3 significant depressive symptoms (including depressed mood, anhedonia, poor appetite, poor sleep, social isolation, feelings of worthlessness, psychomotor changes, irritability, fatigue, and suicidal thoughts).[35]

SUICIDE IN OLDER ADULTS

Older adults in the United States have a high rate of suicide approximately double that of the general American population.[36] Although suicidal behaviors themselves do not seem to increase with advancing age, the rate of completed (successful) suicides increases dramatically. Men (especially whites) predominate in completed suicides among older adults. These elderly men typically select a highly lethal means of suicide, especially gunshot wound to the chest or head (instead of overdose or other less lethal means). African American elders, including men, seem to have a lower rate of suicide. Risk factors for elder suicide include the death of a spouse, living alone, poor perceived health, lack of a confidant, poor sleep, pain, hopelessness, access to a firearm, and other stressful life events. In many cases, elders who commit suicide have visited their primary care physician within a period of a few days before the event. It is therefore important for clinicians to inquire into the question of suicidal ideation. There is no evidence that doing so will awaken such ideas in patients.[36,37]

DIAGNOSTIC EVALUATION

Making the diagnosis of depression in the elderly is accomplished by clinical means, including interview, history, mental status examination, and collateral history. The use of depression scales such as the Patient Health Questionnaire-9, Geriatric Depression Scale, or Beck Depression Inventory may be highly useful to assist with diagnosis and also with tracking symptoms over time.[38,39] Physical and laboratory assessment is important to consider medical factors contributing to depressive symptoms. Laboratory evaluation is useful but often not conclusive, because there is no specific test or biomarker available at present. In many cases, there are multiple factors influencing depressive symptoms, including medical, social, and psychological components. Neuroimaging may be useful in some cases, especially if cerebrovascular disease, cognitive impairment, and dementia are considerations. The diagnostic evaluation should actively consider comorbid medical conditions as well as all medications (including over-the-counter medications). Assessment of cognitive status is also a necessary component of the overall evaluation. Once again, structured interview scales may be invaluable, such as the Montreal Cognitive Assessment, Saint Louis Mental Status, or Mini–Mental State Examination.[40–42] Functional status should include examination of gait and balance, nutritional status (including body weight and weight loss), and other activities of daily living.[24] The patient's living environment as well as family and social support should also be assessed.

TREATMENT OF DEPRESSION IN OLDER ADULTS

Depression in late life is a treatable condition and should be approached with the goal of achieving remission whenever possible. Up to 80% of patients recover from a depressive episode with appropriate therapy.[43] Successful treatment can lead to dramatic improvement in overall function and quality of life, especially in older adult patients. The degree of functional impairment in major depression in older adults is similar to that of a significant medical illness such as heart failure or chronic obstructive pulmonary disease. Treatments for depression include medication therapy, ECT, psychosocial therapies, as well as treatment of associated medical conditions. There is also support for physical activity[44] as well as (especially in seasonal depression) bright light therapy.[45] In regressed medically ill or catatonic patients, stimulants such as methylphenidate or amphetamine preparations may be helpful as stand-alone drugs or in combination with another antidepressant.[46] Stimulants require careful medical evaluation and monitoring. Despite concerns about the potential cardiovascular or psychotomimetic effects of stimulants, these very rarely occur. Instead, suppression of appetite and sleep disturbances are much more common issues. Despite aggressive therapy, however, depression may prove to be treatment resistant in some elders. Older adults are substantially more likely to suffer negative effects of psychiatric medications, which may also require a cautious approach.

There is no single preferred drug for depression in older adults, and a wide variety of medications may be used.[47,48] Selective serotonin reuptake inhibitors (SSRI) are often selected initially for older adults (especially citalopram, escitalopram, and sertraline).[2] Serotonin/norepinephrine reuptake inhibitors (SNRI) and other newer antidepressants (eg, mirtazapine, venlafaxine, desvenlafaxine, duloxetine, and bupropion) may also be used.[49] There is more limited clinical experience with the newest antidepressants with elderly patients (such as vortioxetine, vilazodone, and levomilnacipran). Tricyclic antidepressants and monoamine oxidase inhibitors are much less commonly used in the United States, because of a variety of side-effect and safety issues, but may still be helpful in treatment-resistant cases. The use of polypharmacy in depression has increased greatly, especially multiple antidepressants as well as antipsychotics. Despite these trends, geriatric specialists still seek to limit the number of medications for their patients.[49] In selected cases, antidepressant therapy may be augmented with atypical antipsychotics for agitated, psychotic, or treatment-resistant patients.[50] However, polypharmacy in older patients, especially frail patients, must be approached with an abundance of caution. It is also important to recognize that elders are often underrepresented in clinical trials of antidepressants, especially the types of physically ill, cognitively impaired, or frail patients often encountered in clinical settings.

Extra caution is required in dosing and monitoring for side effects (eg, sedation, ataxia, confusion, cardiovascular effects). The typical course of an antidepressant for an initial episode of major depression that responds to treatment is about 6 to 12 months. This course of treatment may be longer in cases of recurrent depression. Some patients require maintenance medication, especially those with chronic symptoms or frequent recurrences (especially more than 3 lifetime episodes). It may take 4 to 6 weeks to establish the efficacy of a particular antidepressant medication. Medication side effects are always a significant concern when treating elders. The SSRIs are generally regarded as the best tolerated antidepressants, but side effects may occur. They include drug-drug interactions (including cytochrome p-450 effects), hyponatremia, QT interval prolongation, and falling. Other possible side effects include weight loss, sexual dysfunction, agitation, gastrointestinal bleeding, serotonin syndrome, anticholinergic effects, and withdrawal effects.[2]

The response rate to an initial trial of a given antidepressant ranges from 50% to 65%, although there is a lack of data in this area specifically for older adult patients.[51] Multiple trials of medication may produce a higher response rate, although the rate of response to each new antidepressant trial falls after about 2 to 3 medication trials. Increasing the dose of medication beyond the typical level may be considered in cases where no side effects have occurred, especially if partial benefit has been observed. In the case of a treatment failure, a decision must be made whether to switch to a different medication, add a second antidepressant, or add another augmenting agent. Adding a second antidepressant is also often chosen when there is a partial response to the first drug. When adding a second antidepressant, an agent from a different pharmacologic class is usually selected. When switching to a new antidepressant, clinicians have historically also selected a drug from a new class. However, it now seems clear that even when a drug from a particular class has failed, the likelihood of success with a drug from the same class or a different class is about equal. Historically, buspirone, thyroid medications, and lithium were among the typical selections for augmentation. However, today it is more common to add an atypical antipsychotic such as aripiprazole or quetiapine, typically in low doses. If polypharmacy is considered, the potential harmful effects must be weighed against the possibility of boosting response rate. Some common mistakes in antidepressant therapy include reliance on antianxiety or sleeping medications (especially benzodiazepines), excessive polypharmacy, inadequate dose or duration of medication trial, and giving up too soon. Genomic testing for antidepressants has recently been made available, attempting to screen patients for any genetic condition that might have an impact on the utility or side-effect profile of several different medications. However, the clinical utility of this approach, especially in older patients, is not yet clear.

Anxiety symptoms and disorders commonly cooccur with depression among elderly patients. In the past, benzodiazepines or other sedative hypnotics have been widely prescribed. However, an abundance of evidence is now available highlighting the potential risks of benzodiazepines and related medications. These risks include sedation, falling, accidents, cognitive clouding, increased risk of developing dementia, and others. The use of benzodiazepines should be limited. A common clinical dilemma is the case of a depressed or anxious older adult patient who has been taking a benzodiazepine for several years at the time of evaluation. Such a patient is very likely to have both physical and psychological dependence on the medication and be very reluctant to discontinue it. The best approach is usually to establish a strong therapeutic alliance with the patient, reassure them that their concerns are important, seek to address the symptoms in alternate ways, and very gradually wean the medication over a period of months.

ELECTROCONVULSIVE THERAPY

ECT can be used safely and effectively in elders for severe or treatment-resistant depression, despite the controversies that have existed about this treatment over a period of decades.[52,53] Treatment resistance in this case may be defined as a failure of at least 2 well-conducted trials of medication therapy. A very large number of older patients would be classified into this category, but in clinical practice, only the most severe cases are generally considered for ECT. Another group of good candidates for ECT includes those patients who have responded well to ECT in the past. In such cases, it is often prudent to consider ECT early in the course of a relapse rather than waiting for multiple medication failures. ECT typically involves a series of roughly 6 to 12 treatments over a period of several weeks, although the number of treatments is determined by the patient's response. ECT may sometimes be effective in treatment-resistant cases of depression even when multiple medications have failed. The overall response rate in ECT is much higher than with medications, in the 80% to 90% range. ECT is the treatment of choice for most patients with catatonia and is also a highly effective therapy for psychotic depression. Relative to medications, it has a much more rapid rate of response. Despite these relative advantages, ECT is not a permanent cure for depression. It is best regarded as a potent treatment of a given episode. It also has several drawbacks, including the need for general anesthesia, and the risk of short-term cognitive impairment. Although ECT may sometimes be conducted on an outpatient basis, many elders with medical or frailty issues require psychiatric hospitalization for the treatment. Despite substantial literature on ECT in the elderly, there are very few rigorous studies, and ECT does not lend itself to placebo controlled trials, the gold standard of outcome measures.[54] Nevertheless, the available evidence strongly suggests that ECT for elders has an excellent safety and effectiveness record, especially considering the consequences of unremitting depression. In selected patients, maintenance ECT may be advisable to maintain a state of remission. Maintenance ECT is usually considered in cases where there is an established tendency toward rapid relapse into depression. Occasionally, ECT may be used in other conditions, including mania and catatonic syndromes not clearly associated with depression (such as neuroleptic malignant syndrome, Parkinson disease, or dementia). Alternatives to ECT have been introduced in recent years, including repetitive transcranial stimulation (rTMS). rTMS is a therapy for treatment-resistant depression involving repetitively stimulating a portion of the frontal cortex with a powerful magnetic coil. The treatment is performed on an outpatient basis over a period of weeks, typically involving roughly 25 to 30 sessions. No anesthesia is required; no seizure is induced, and there is no cognitive impairment associated with the therapy. The overall success rates for this treatment are lower than for ECT (for all patients, about 50%–60%), although patient acceptance and tolerance are high. The long-term effects of rTMS on the course of depression are not yet clear. Experience with rTMS for elders so far is somewhat limited, and the results appear to be mixed with a suggestion that elders as a group may not respond as well as younger patients.[55]

PSYCHOSOCIAL THERAPIES

A variety of psychological factors may play a role in elder depression. These psychological issues may include grief and loss, widowhood, the "empty nest," retirement, pain, and illness. Regrets experienced over a lifetime may play a role in an older patient. Fears of financial problems, dependency, loneliness, existential issues of aging, and mortality are also potent issues. A belief once existed that older adult patients were not suitable candidates for psychotherapy. Experience has shown that a variety of approaches that have been developed for late life psychotherapy may be helpful for depression. Supportive psychotherapy focuses on ego support, practical advice, medication compliance, psychoeducation, activities, and maintaining a hopeful attitude. Cognitive behavioral therapy (CBT) is a structured, agenda-based therapy focusing on identifying and modifying self-defeating patterns of thought and behavior in the present, rather than focusing on the unconscious or the distant past.[56,57] The patient is encouraged to acquire skills in therapy that may be useful in addressing depressive symptoms directly and serve to limit the risk of relapse. Modifications of CBT may be required, especially for the frail, physically ill, or cognitively impaired older adult patient.[58,59] The therapist may need to adapt the pace and process of therapy in the case of loss of attention, stamina, and slowed thinking. The therapist may have to be more active and provide sufficient energy to engage the elderly patient. The family often needs to be involved to a greater extent than in nongeriatric patients. The typical here-and-now focus of CBT may be relaxed to allow for life review and existential tasks. Homework assignments, a typical element of CBT, may be simple and immediate. Aspects of CBT with elders may include behavioral activation, positive reinforcement, identifying strengths, and realistic coping with loss or illness.

Interpersonal therapy involves a focus on roles and role transitions and has been much discussed but little used in older depressive outside of academic centers.[60] Problem-solving therapy is a relatively new and promising therapy that focuses on helping depressed patients recognize key life problems and develop and implement practical plans to address them.[61,62]

BIPOLAR DEPRESSION IN OLDER ADULTS

Bipolar disorder typically has its onset in the late adolescent or young adult years. However, the disorder is a life-long condition of remitting and relapsing episodes of mood disorder. Bipolar disorder is unfortunately associated with a high level of mortality and a shortened lifespan by up to 2 decades in the United States. Nevertheless, although younger patients are more commonly discussed in the literature, older patients with bipolar depression are relatively frequently encountered in geriatric practice. There are few guidelines for treating these patients. They may present with mixed or irritable symptoms or episodes rather than the typical highs or lows, and well or euthymic periods may be briefer. Cognitive impairment and a high degree of medical morbidity appear to be common in this population. Psychotic depression and catatonia also appear to be overrepresented. The usual mood stabilizers may be useful, such as divalproex, carbamazepine, and lithium, but may be more difficult to manage and may require lower doses and blood levels. Anecdotal evidence suggests that antidepressants are more commonly used in this group than in younger bipolars, and may be better tolerated.

SUMMARY

Depression is not a normal part of aging and should be regarded as a serious, disabling medical disorder. There are a growing number of cases of late life depression owing to a growth in the at-risk population, although an earlier belief that depression increases with age appears to be incorrect. The prevalence of depression in older American adults appears to be similar to other age groups. A major focus of the field is to understand how depression among older adults intersects with grief, medical illnesses, and dementia. The illness is recognized as heterogeneous, and various diagnostic constructs may be applied. These constructs include major depression, minor depression, persistent depressive disorder, late life onset depression, vascular depression, and depression of AD, among others. Suicide is an important consideration in the management of elder depression, especially among older white men; an active approach by clinicians is warranted. Pharmacotherapy is important, especially with the SSRIs and SNRIs. ECT remains an important option, especially for catatonic, psychotic, or treatment-resistant cases of elder depression, but the role of rTMS is still being clarified. Psychotherapy is an important and often overlooked treatment option for geriatric depression, and our knowledge in this area has grown greatly in recent years, particularly for CBT. Depression in the elderly should be viewed as a treatable condition. Successful treatment may greatly improve the patient's function and quality of life.

REFERENCES

1. Casey DA. Depression in the elderly: a review and update. Asia Pac Psychiatr 2011;4:160–7.
2. Blazer D. Depression in late life: review and commentary. Focus 2009;7:118–36 [reprinted from J Gerontol A Biol Sci Med Sci 2003;58A(3):249–65].

3. Alexopolous GS, Kelly RE. Research advances in geriatric depression. World Psychiatry 2009;8(3):140–9.

4. Day JC. U.S. Bureau of the Census: population projections in the United States, by age, sex, race, and Hispanic origin, 1993-2050. Current population reports. Washington, DC: U.S. Government Printing Office; 1996. p. 25–1104.

5. American Psychiatric Association: Diagnostic and Statistical Manual of Mental Disorders (DSM-5). 5th Edition. Arlington (VA): American Psychiatric Association; 2013. p. 160–8.

6. Steffens DC, Skoog I, Norton MC, et al. Prevalence of depression and its treatment in an elderly population. Arch Gen Psychiatry 2000;57:601–7.

7. Yohannes AM, Baldwin RC, Connolly MJ. Prevalence of depression and anxiety symptoms in elderly patients admitted in post-acute intermediate care. Int J Geriatr Psychiatry 2008;23:1141–7.

8. Jongenelis K, Pot AM, Eisses AM, et al. Prevalence and risk indicators of depression in elderly nursing home patients: the AGED study. J Affect Disord 2004; 83(2–3):135–42.

9. Lyness JM, Heo M, Datto CJ, et al. Outcomes of minor and subsyndromal depression among elderly patients in primary care settings. Ann Intern Med 2006;144:496–504.

10. Vahia IV, Meeks TW, Thompson WK, et al. Subthreshold depression and successful aging in older women. Am J Geriatr Psychiatry 2010;18(3):212–20.

11. Williams JW, Barrett J, Oxman T, et al. Treatment of dysthymia and minor depression in primary care. J Am Med Assoc 2000;284(12):1519–26.

12. Cohen CI, Magai C, Yaffee R, et al. Racial differences in syndromal and subsyndromal depression in an older urban population. Psychiatr Serv 2005;56(12):1556–63.

13. Alexopolous GS. The vascular depression hypothesis: 10 years later. Biol Psychiatry 2006;60:1304–5.

14. Sneed JR, Culang-Reinlieb ME. The vascular depression hypothesis: an update. Am J Geriatr Psychiatry 2011;19(2):99–103.

15. Beck AT, Alford BA. Depression: causes and treatment. 2nd edition. Philadelphia: University of Pennsylvania Press; 2009. p. 77.

16. Gallo JJ, Rabins PV. Depression without sadness: alternative presentations of depression in late life. Am Fam Physician 1999;60:820–6.

17. Evans M, Mottram P. Diagnosis of depression in elderly patients. Adv Psychiatr Treat 2000;6:49–56.

18. Robertson RG, Montagnini M. Geriatric failure to thrive. Am Fam Physician 2004; 70(2):343–50.

19. Adams KB. Depressive symptoms, depletion, or developmental change? Withdrawal, apathy, and lack of vigor on the geriatric depression scale. Gerontologist 2001;41(6):768–77.

20. Kennedy G. Advances in the treatment of late-life psychotic depression. Prim Psychiatr 2004;15(7):27–9.

21. Meyers BS, Flint AJ, Rothschild AJ, et al. A double-blind randomized controlled trial of olanzapine plus sertraline vs olanzapine plus placebo for psychotic depression. Arch Gen Psychiatry 2009;66(8):838–47.

22. Steffens DC. Imaging and genetics advances in understanding geriatric depression. Neuropsychopharmacology 2010;35:348–9.

23. Casey DA. Management of the patient in geriatric psychiatry. In: Tasman A, Kay J, Lieberman J, et al, editors. Psychiatry. 3rd edition. Chichester (England): Wiley; 2008. p. 2549–62.

24. Charlson M, Peterson JC. Medical comorbidity and late life depression: what is known and what are the unmet needs? Biol Psychiatry 2002;52:226–35.
25. Noel PH, Williams JW, Unutzer J, et al. Depression and comorbid illness in elderly primary care patients: impact on multiple domains of health status and well-being. Ann Fam Med 2004;2(6):555–62.
26. Bigger JT, Glassman AH. The American Heart Association science advisory on depression and coronary heart disease: an exploration of the issues raised. Cleve Clin J Med 2010;77(Suppl 3):S12–9.
27. Pitt B, Deldin PJ. Depression and cardiovascular disease: have a happy day-just smile! Eur Heart J 2010;31(9):1036–7.
28. Cho HJ, Lavretsky H, Olmstead R, et al. Prior depression history and deterioration of physical health in community-dwelling older adults-a prospective cohort study. Am J Geriatr Psychiatry 2010;18(5):442–51.
29. Luber MP, Meyers BS, Williams-Russo PG, et al. Depression and service utilization in elderly primary care patients. Am J Geriatr Psychiatry 2001;9(2):169–76.
30. Dhondt T, Beekman AT, Deeg DJ, et al. Iatrogenic depression in the elderly: results from a community based study in the Netherlands. Soc Psychiatry Psychiatr Epidemiol 2002;37(8):393–8.
31. Beal E. Dementia: depression and dementia. Nat Rev Neurol 2010;6(9):470.
32. Dotson VM, Beydoun MA, Zonderman AB. Recurrent depressive symptoms and the incidence of dementia and mild cognitive impairment. Neurology 2010;75:27–34.
33. Saczynski JS, Beiser A, Seshadri S, et al. Depressive symptoms and risk of dementia. Neurology 2010;75:35–41.
34. Wells CE. Pseudodementia. Am J Psychiatry 1979;136:895–900.
35. Rosenberg PB, Onyike C, Katz IR, et al. Clinical application of operationalized criteria for "Depression of Alzheimer's disease". Int J Geriatr Psychiatry 2005; 20(2):119–27.
36. Casey DA. Suicide in the elderly: a two-year study of data from death certificates. South Med J 1991;84(10):1185–7.
37. Conwell Y, Thompson C. Suicidal behavior in elders. Psychiatr Clin North Am 2008;31(2):333–56.
38. Yesavage JA, Brink TL, Rose TL, et al. Development and validation of a geriatric depression screening scale: a preliminary report. J Psychiatr Res 1982–1983; 17(1):37–49.
39. Phelan E, Williams B, Meeker K, et al. A study of the diagnostic accuracy of the PHQ-9 in primary care elderly. BMC Fam Pract 2010;11:63.
40. Folstein MF, Folstein SE, McHugh PR. "Mini-mental state": a practical method for grading the cognitive state of patients for the clinician. J Psychiatr Res 1975; 12(3):189–98.
41. Nasreddine ZS, Phillips NA, Bedirian V, et al. The Montreal Cognitive Assessment, MoCA: a brief screening tool for mild cognitive impairment. J Am Geriatr Soc 2005;53(4):695–9.
42. Tariq SH, Tumosa N, Chibnall JT, et al. Comparison of the Saint Louis University mental status examination and the mini-mental state examination for detecting dementia and mild neurocognitive disorder-a pilot study. Am J Geriatr Psychiatry 2006;14(11):900–10.
43. Reynolds E, Frank C, Perel J, et al. Combined pharmacotherapy and psychotherapy in the acute and continuation treatment of elderly patients with recurrent major depression: a preliminary report. Am J Psychiatry 1992;149:1687–92.
44. Sjoesten N, Kivel SL. The effects of physical exercise on depressive symptoms among the aged: a systematic review. Int J Geriatr Psychiatry 2006;21(5):410–8.

45. Lieverse R, Van Someren EJ, Nielen MM, et al. Bright light treatment in elderly patients with non-seasonal major depressive disorder. A randomized placebo controlled trial. Arch Gen Psychiatry 2011;68(1):61–70.
46. Prowler ML, Weiss D, Caroff SN. Treatment of catatonia with methylphenidate in an elderly patient with depression. Psychosomatics 2010;51(1):74–6.
47. Salzman C, Wong E, Wright BC. Drug and ECT treatment of depression in the elderly, 1996-2001: a literature review. Biol Psychiatry 2002;52(3):265–84.
48. Alexopoulos GS. Depression in the elderly. Lancet 2005;365(9475):1961–70.
49. Alexopoulos GS, Katz IR, Reynolds CF, et al. The expert consensus guideline series. Pharmacotherapy of depressive disorders in older patients. Postgrad Med 2001;Spec No Pharmacotherapy: special edition:1–86.
50. Alexopoulos GS. Pharmacotherapy for late-life depression. J Clin Psychiatry 2011;72(1):e04.
51. Taylor WD, Doraiswamy PM. A systematic review of antidepressant placebo-controlled trials for geriatric depression: limitations of current data and directions for the future. Neuropsychopharmacology 2004;29:2285–99.
52. Casey DA, Davis MH. Electroconvulsive therapy in the very old. Gen Hosp Psychiatry 1996;18:436–9.
53. Flint AJ, Gagnon N. Effective use of electroconvulsive therapy in late-life depression. Can J Psychiatry 2002;47(8):734–41.
54. van der Wurff FB, Stek ML, Hoogendijk WJ, et al. The efficacy and safety of ECT in depressed older adults, a literature review. Int J Geriatr Psychiatry 2003;18: 894–904.
55. Jalenques I, Legrand G, Vaille-Perret E, et al. Therapeutic efficacy and safety of repetitive transcranial magnetic stimulation in depressions of the elderly: a review. Encephale 2009;36(Suppl 2):D105–18 [in French].
56. Laidlaw K, Thompson LW, Gallagher-Thompson D, et al. Cognitive behaviour therapy with older people. West Sussex (United Kingdom): Wiley; 2003. p. 232.
57. Gallagher-Thompson D, Thompson LW. Treating later life depression. A cognitive-behavioral approach, therapist guide. New York: Oxford University Press; 2010. p. 241.
58. Evans C. Cognitive-behavioural therapy with older people. Adv Psychiatr Treat 2007;13(2):111–8.
59. Casey DA, Grant RW. Cognitive therapy with geropsychiatric inpatients. In: Wright JH, Thase ME, Beck AT, et al, editors. The cognitive milieu: inpatient applications of cognitive therapy. New York: Guilford Publications; 1992. p. 295–314.
60. Miller MD. Using interpersonal therapy (IPT) with older adults today and tomorrow: a review of the literature and new developments. Curr Psychiatry Rep 2008;10(1): 16–22.
61. Alexopoulos GS, Raue P, Arean P. Problem-solving therapy vs. supportive therapy in geriatric major depression with executive dysfunction. Am J Geriatr Psychiatry 2003;11(1):46–52.
62. Arean P, Raue P, Mackin RS, et al. Problem solving therapy and supportive therapy for older adults with major depression and executive dysfunction. Am J Psychiatry 2010;167(11):1391–8.

Managing Polypharmacy in the 15-Minute Office Visit

Demetra Antimisiaris, PharmD, BCGP, FASCP[a,b,c,]*, Timothy Cutler, PharmD, BCGP[d]

KEYWORDS

- Polypharmacy • Medication reconciliation • Potentially inappropriate medications
- Beers criteria • Morisky scale • Geriatric syndromes
- Comprehensive medication management • Drug interactions

KEY POINTS

- The prevalence of polypharmacy is significant and growing, with the United States leading the world in medication per capita use. Older adults live with polypharmacy due to high chronic and acute disease burden.
- Polypharmacy (medication management) skills are essential when caring for older adults and can offer improved quality measure outcomes and improved reimbursements.
- The health care system and multiple providers contribute to the syndrome of polypharmacy. At minimum, a thorough medication reconciliation and medication management session should be performed at least annually.
- Proactive implementation of a systematic polypharmacy management program (despite the 15-minute office visit rush) is preferable to reactive management of sometimes serious medication-related problems.
- Efficient involvement of the patient, the office team, and community resources can result in improved medication management and outcomes.

INTRODUCTION

The American Board of Internal Medicine Foundation launched an initiative called Choosing Wisely, with the goal of advancing dialogue on wasteful or unnecessary medical tests, treatments, and procedures (American Medical Board Foundation. Choosing Wisely. Available at http://www.choosingwisely.org). The Choosing

This article originally appeared in *Primary Care Clinics: Clinics in Office Practice*, Volume 44, Issue 3, September 2017.

The authors have nothing to disclosures.

[a] Pharmacy and Medication Management Program, Department of Pharmacology and Toxicology, University of Louisville, 501 East Broadway, Suite 240, Louisville, KY 40202, USA; [b] Department of Neurology, University of Louisville, 501 East Broadway, Suite 240, Louisville, KY 40202, USA; [c] Department of Family Medicine and Geriatrics, University of Louisville, 501 East Broadway, Suite 240, Louisville, KY 40202, USA; [d] Department of Clinical Pharmacy, UCSF School of Pharmacy, 533 Parnassus Avenue U585, UCSF POBox 0622, San Francisco, CA 94117, USA
* Corresponding author. Department of Family Medicine and Geriatrics, University of Louisville, 501 East Broadway, Suite 240, Louisville, KY 40202.
E-mail address: demetra.antimisiaris@louisville.edu

Wisely campaign asked national organizations representing medical specialists to identify areas of potential waste and the American Geriatrics Society in 2013 released their Choosing Wisely list of 10 things clinicians and patients should question; 7 of the 10 Choosing Wisely recommendations pertain to medication use.[1]

The need for the care of older adults has increased over the past several years, especially as it relates to the use of medications in older adults. From the years 1998 to 2008, the overall rate of office visits for those over age 65 increased by 13%. For those visits where medications were prescribed or continued, patients over age 65 had the highest increase in visits (31%) compared with any other age group.[2] In the new era of quality measure reporting and incentives, management of medications in the elderly has become an important element of primary care. For example, the Physician Quality Reporting System and the Medicare Access and CHIP Reauthorization Act implemented by the Centers for Medicare and Medicaid Services list several measures that evaluate appropriate medication management as an integral part of outcomes ranging from management of neuropsychiatric symptoms of dementia, plan of care for falls, urinary incontinence plan of care, diabetes control, statin therapy for prevention of cardiovascular disease, and medication reconciliation postdischarge. Failure to achieve quality thresholds results in lower Medicare payments to individual and group practices.

Any symptom in an elderly patient should be considered a medication related problem until proved otherwise
—Gurwitz J, Monane M, Monane S, and Avorn J. Brown University Long-Term
Care Quality Letter, 2001.[3]

The challenges of appropriate management of medications in older adults can be broken down into the following areas: multimorbidity, polypharmacy PIMs in the elderly, underuse of medications, and adherence and access to medications. There are several challenges specific to primary care providers (PCPs) when managing these issues in older adults, which include the brevity of the typical office visit; medically complex patients; multiple specialists who contribute to a patient's overall polypharmacy; frequent hospitalizations and transitions of care; lack of high-quality evidence to guide prescribing for older adults, in particular the old-old, who are typically over 80 years of age; and the fact that evidence-based guidelines rely on clinical trials that typically exclude multimorbid and frail older adults.[4–7]

Polypharmacy is traditionally defined in the literature as the use of 5 or more chronic medications, the use of inappropriate medications, or medications that are not clinically warranted.[8] Historically, the 15-minute office visit consists of approximately 7 minutes dedicated to establishment of the problem, 3.5 minutes to work on the problem, and 3.5 minutes dedicated to medications.[4] Patients living with polypharmacy do not have much opportunity to have their overall medication needs addressed in a clinic visit. In the era of quality measure reimbursement, these challenges also present an opportunity to demonstrate improvement of outcomes and leveraging quality-based reimbursements through proactive attention to management of polypharmacy.

There is increasing evidence of the value, decreased morbidity, and mortality as well as return on investment when focused medication management occurs.[9–15] The intent of this article is to provide some strategies PCPs to provide overall polypharmacy management for the increasing cohort of older adult patients expected in the coming years.

ACHIEVING OPTIMAL POLYPHARMACY MANAGEMENT IN THE OLDER ADULT
Focus on Monitoring Medication Use

Older adults live with multiple chronic conditions, underlying incidents of acute medical and functional problems, which leads to multiple transitions of care. Multimorbidity and transitions of care leads to polypharmacy, which is considered a geriatric syndrome. Geriatric syndromes are problems that are highly prevalent in older adults, especially frail older adults. Geriatric syndromes do not refer to an organic disease but multifactorial issues involved with multiple problems, leading to added impairment and negative impact on quality of life. Examples of geriatric syndromes include but are not limited to dizziness, cognitive impairment, delirium, falls, frailty, syncope, urinary incontinence, and polypharmacy. A core principle of the management of polypharmacy in older adults is avoidance of PIMS. Ultimately, determination of whether a medication is inappropriate or not is highly individualized and often circumstantial as well. A medication that is inappropriate now, for example highly elevated carbidopa-levodopa doses in a patient long term on high doses, may become appropriate again after a carbidopa-levodopa high-dose holiday. Medications that are considered potentially inappropriate in general can be found in 2 established resources that serve as guidance on PIMS in older adults. These 2 resources are the Beers criteria and the START and STOPP criteria.[16,17] The use of the Beers criteria and START and STOPP criteria is discussed later.

Polypharmacy and the health care system: the care of older adults is typically provided by multiple specialists, in addition to PCPs, as well as several ancillary care providers. A silo effect can occur, where each care provider works on a specific problem without ever having an opportunity to communicate or discuss with the other providers. Adding to the silo effect are the various care settings that older adults frequent, such as hospitals, assisted living residences, nursing homes, postdischarge rehabilitation facilities, adult day care, and more. The complexity and velocity of care changes multimorbid older adults live with lead to a dearth of opportunities to perform needed comprehensive medication reconciliation (CMR), leading to unchecked polypharmacy and undesirable outcomes.[18] Each transition of care should warrant a CMR, and even when a CMR is just performed at least annually, up to 90% of patients have some form of medication-related problem identified.[19] CMR and comprehensive medication management (CMM) are challenging to fit into a busy primary care (or specialty) office practice. Medicare offers an annual CMM for beneficiaries through Medicare D. Medication therapy management service is provided through a Medicare patient's pharmacy benefits manager and patients can be referred for a CMM by helping them to contact their pharmacy benefits manager and be assigned a consultant. There are innovative models, particularly associated with patient-centered medical home models, which provide the operationalization methods (billing models) to provide improved CMR and CMM in the office practice.[20,21]

One immediate means of implementing improved medication management is to focus on monitoring and pharmacovigilance. There is evidence that medication monitoring is an often-missed opportunity to prevent adverse drug events (ADEs).[22] The major factors leading to ADEs in ambulatory community-dwelling older adults have been identified as rooted in problems with monitoring, prescribing, and adherence. Monitoring is involved in approximately 60% of ADEs, prescribing involved in 58%, and adherence involved in 60% (more than 1 of these factors could contribute to each incident).[22]

Two major studies of older adults evaluating emergency department visits and hospitalizations for ADEs found that drugs, such as digoxin, warfarin, insulins, oral antiplatelet agents, and oral hypoglycemic agents, were responsible for a majority of hospitalizations (39% and 67%, respectively) and PIMs included on the Beers list were responsible for only 1.2% of hospitalizations. Digoxin, warfarin, insulins, oral antiplatelets, and oral hypoglycemic medications were 35 times more likely to result in hospitalization than medications considered potentially inappropriate for older adults.[23,24] Although the Beers list of PIMs in the elderly is important, the medications consistently found to result in older adults' hospital visits are medications that are commonly in use, the monitoring parameters of which are well known. These studies support the idea that potentially missed monitoring of routine, daily use medications, for chronic disease can result in serious medication misadventure in the elderly. Additional evidence supporting the need for appropriate medication monitoring includes a systematic review, which evaluates preventable ADEs in ambulatory care patients, and found that 45% of preventable adverse drug reactions were due to inadequate monitoring and 16% due to ignoring or missing a clinical or laboratory result.[25]

Because the effort required to have an impact on patient adherence is labor intensive and challenging, PCPs working toward more effective medication monitoring may be more easily achieved than working on adherence[26] (CMM consults through Medicare D can provide a means of working on adherence as well as peer disease support groups and midlevel providers). Monitoring medication use in the office practice is achievable when a systematic approach is implemented, such as that used to monitor international normalization ratio for persons receiving warfarin.

Appropriate monitoring of medication use requires setting up a system to provide periodic interval monitoring for each medication a patient is using. Such a system might include assigning tracking of monitoring to medical staff, because sometimes complex medication use tracks 20 or more medications for 1 patient. Similar systems are often used for international normalization ratio tracking in patients using warfarin. Alternately, electronic records could be designed to track missed monitoring. Besides tracking intervals of monitoring for each medication, a clinic team could perform other tasks, such as database scanning for recommended monitoring appropriate for each drug and drug interaction evaluation. Clerkship students, midlevel providers, or other members of the primary care team can perform this routine work as well.

People often think of drug monitoring as making sure the laboratory monitoring associated with a drug is completed. But other important forms of monitoring include following drug monograph recommendations to track and document common adverse events for each medication, common medication–disease adverse events, drug-drug interactions, and monitoring renal, hepatic, and cytochrome enzyme clearance interactions.

Lastly, a commonly overlooked form of monitoring is monitoring for efficacy. If efficacy is nonexistent, then a medication should be discontinued from use (**Box 1**).

Algorithms and processes for monitoring appropriateness and need of medication use in older adults have been created and can be useful in developing a systematic approach to medication use monitoring[27,28] (see algorithm by Garfinkle and colleagues, referenced in *UptoDate*).[29]

Heightened efforts to monitor drug use would work toward decreasing the incidence of overlooked pharmacovigilance, thus preventing emergency department visits and hospitalizations.[30,31]

Deprescribing and Prescribing of Omitted Therapies

Deprescribing has been demonstrated as a useful tool in optimization of functional status and diminishing medication-related problem risks, where the number of medications taken by a patient is the single most important predictor of inappropriate

---

Box 1
Medication monitoring check list

- Efficacy—if not efficacious, consider deprescribing.

- Laboratory monitoring—track, follow-up, and implement at appropriate intervals.

- Drug-drug interactions—run a drug interaction checker periodically and document presence or absence of drug interactions.

- Drug-disease interactions

- Monitor renal, hepatic clearance.

- Keep aware of cytochrome enzyme clearance interactions—for example, a course of fluconazole can cause phenytoin to become toxic.

---

medication use.[32] Deprescribing is the process of stopping or tapering medications to minimize inappropriate medication use or polypharmacy. The goal is to target one at a time and to avoid changing too many items at once or abruptly.

Consideration of deprescribing of a medication: look for medications that have no valid reason for being used; evaluate the overall risk of drug-induced harm; assess current or future benefit versus risk; prioritize discontinuation and consider removal of medications with lowest benefit to heightened harm risk first; and implement a plan to discontinue (perhaps a taper) and monitor follow-up. Typically, the medications that have no accompanying diagnosis, problems, or obvious reason for use are there because they are treating underappreciated side effects of other medications. It is best to strive to manage the side effects of offending agents first by optimizing dose or selection of another medication for the problem rather than making the drug tolerable by treating the side effect.

Scan for PIMs for elderly patients by consulting criteria regarding PIM and appropriate medication use in older adults, such as the Beers criteria and START and STOPP criteria. These criteria also present evidence and expert opinion regarding underprescribed medications that should be used in the elderly (ie, warfarin in atrial fibrillation patients who fall; although is counterintuitive, the supporting evidence is presented).[16,17]

Avoid the Prescribing Cascade

Systematic medication monitoring should accompany vigilance in avoiding the prescribing cascade. The prescribing cascade occurs when a medication is used to treat the side effect of another medication (**Fig. 1**). For most cases, the prescribing cascade dynamic is undesirable but sometimes it is intentional. Examples of prescribing a medication to treat the side effects of another medication are (1) a patient taking antipsychotic agents resulting in extrapyramidal symptoms, and anticholinergic agents are prescribed to treat the extrapyramidal symptoms when the benefit of antipsychotic agent use outweighs the risks, and (2) the use of a stimulant laxative for patients receiving chronic opioids.

Individualization of Medication Use

An important consideration in the care of older adults is the need for individualization of care due to the heterogeneous health status of persons aged 65 and older. Most single-disease practice guidelines do not include evidence derived from multimorbidity patients or persons with advanced age.[33] With age, patients become physiologically and functionally very different from one another due to chronic disease and

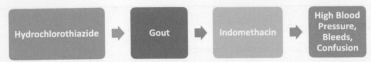

Fig. 1. Prescribing CASCADE-In this example, hydrochlorothiazide used for hypertension, eventually leads to gout, which is treated with indomethacin, which becomes the cause of dangerously high blood pressure, nose bleeds, and confusion (not recommended for older adults per Beers criteria, yet a drug of choice for gout treatment). The prescribing CASCADE described here is a real case, resolved permanently by substitution of hydrochlorothiazide with low dose amlodipine.

individual morbidity burdens, which leads to individualized life expectancies and physiologic reserve. The physiologic changes that occur with age, such as diminished renal function and increased percent body fat with decreased percent body water, have an impact on the way medications perform pharmacokinetically, and altered pharmacodynamic response is influenced by these pharmacokinetic changes as well as underlying physiologic pathologies, such as impaired baroreceptor response. Age is only a surrogate marker for many of the factors to consider in choosing treatment options. There are people in their early 60s with serious debility and others near 90 who are busy climbing mountains. The Food and Drug Administration (FDA) recently mandated increased inclusion of more subjects over 65 years of age in clinical trials, yet most trials do not reflect the actual proportion of older adults living with the disease for which the medication is being tested.[34] The effects of comorbidities on disease-specific outcomes are inadequately studied in chronic disease trials from which clinical guidelines are derived.[35,36]

The cornerstone of treatment recommendations are chronic disease guidelines and other disease-specific guidelines resulting in the use multiple medications, especially in those with multiple conditions. The ability to sustain high drug burden and other interventions is relative to factors, such as frailty, physiologic reserve, and total disease burden.[37–39] Conversely, there is the question of the impact of medications on functional status.[40] Polypharmacy resulting from multiple providers following disease practice guidelines, resulting in untested combinations of medications, can be associated with suboptimal functional status and negative outcomes.[41–44] That said, robust older adults who are living with minimal chronic disease burden and minimal functional impairment can benefit from long-term disease prevention just as a younger person can.

Application of clinical practice guidelines to the older adult patient requires special assessment and consideration: Are patients robust or frail? What is their functional status? Is the current functional status temporary or long term? How heavy is their comorbidity and geriatric syndrome burden? What are their preferences and goals of care? How does a patient's quality of life interplay with these considerations? Is the patient able to adhere to treatment? What are the risks versus benefits of treatment? What is the time horizon to benefit versus patient's life expectancy?

Consider the recent changes in the United States guidelines for diabetes, lipids, and hypertension. All of them have added a statement of individualization of care for those over 80 years of age, and the statin use guidelines have explicitly included consideration of 10-year cardiovascular risk in determining medication use choices.[45–47] These major chronic disease guidelines have acknowledged that application of the evidence, such as time to benefit, time to harm, and other parameters, are applied differently to individuals outside the (younger and less medically complex) study population, such as some older adults.

The American Geriatrics Society Expert Panel on the Care of Older Adults with Multimorbidity[48] recommends a stepwise approach. The approach explains an algorithm that includes patient's primary concern, consideration of relevant evidence, prognosis, interactions with and among treatments and conditions, benefits versus harms, communication, and reassessment for alignment with preferences, feasibility, adherence, and benefit at selected intervals. For some patients, careful consideration of multimorbidity effects on treatments can have a marked impact on medication management decisions. In addition to the American Geriatrics Society approach, a classic algorithm to help determine appropriateness of medication use is the Medication Appropriateness Index, illustrated in **Box 2**.

Lastly, after ensuring a patient's understanding of conditions, medications, and risks versus benefits, the importance of finding out if the patient wants to take the medications being prescribed or recommended to take should not be overlooked. For a comprehensive online review of person-centered medication use optimization, refer to the British National Institute for Health and Care Excellence guideline.[49]

As for medication dosing, the rule of thumb in terms of titrating medication dose is "start low and go slow." Although medications typically are accompanied by target dosing, for the frail elderly, targeting the minimum effective dose is a safer approach.

Verification of appropriate renal dose adjustment should be checked for each medication an older adult patient is taking. The renal dose adjustment should be made using the Cockroft-Gault equation for estimated creatinine clearance for 2 reasons: first, the Cockroft-Gault method is the FDA standard by which dose recommendations in the drug monographs are reported (thus to use another equation would be like comparing apples to oranges), and second, the Cockroft-Gault equation underestimates renal clearance compared with the estimated glomerular filtration rate, Modificaiton of Diet in Renal Disease, or gold standard of 24-hour urine collection. Underestimation of renal function is typically safer for older adults regarding renal dose adjustment for medications. The Cockroft-Gault equation is easily found in point-of-care applications, such as Epocrates, Lexicomp, and online support sites,

---

Box 2
Medication appropriateness index

1. Is there an indication for the drug?

2. Is the medication effective for the condition?

3. Is the dosage correct?

4. Are the directions correct?

5. Are the directions practical?

6. Are there clinically significant drug-drug interactions?

7. Are there clinically significant drug-disease/condition interactions?

8. Is there unnecessary duplication with other drugs?

9. Is the duration of therapy acceptable?

10. Is this drug the least expensive alternative compared with others of equal usefulness?

From Hanlon JT, Schmader KE, Samsa GP, et al. A method for assessing drug therapy appropriateness. J Clin Epidemiol 1992;45(10):1045–51; with permission.

such as GlobalRPh or National Kidney Foundation. Typically, height, weight, and serum creatinine level are needed at hand to use these calculators. If there is not a serum creatinine level, for persons over 65 year of age, a minimum creatinine clearance can be estimated using serum creatinine = 1 mg/dL. In persons over 65, even if the serum creatinine is less than 1 mg/dL, clinical medication consultants typically round up to 1 mg/dL because most persons over 65 have some degree of sarcopenia, which can cause misleading creatinine levels for estimating renal clearance. Also, it is important to use stable serum creatinine levels. Much like blood pressure, one reading may reflect a transient condition due to medication use, dehydration, or some other renal accident.[50]

IMPLEMENTATION OF POLYPHARMACY MANAGEMENT IN THE 15-MINUTE OFFICE VISIT

It is important to recognize that optimal polypharmacy management does not occur in 15 minutes. Proactively and systematically, however, checking off some of the elements of optimal polypharmacy management during each visit and repeating periodically (annually perhaps) is preferable to addressing polypharmacy when problems arise **(Fig. 2)**.

Medication Reconciliation

Medication reconciliation is typically defined as getting the most accurate list of medications a patient is using. Appropriate medication reconciliation involves patient and caregiver interviews, lists from health records, pharmacy records, hospitalization

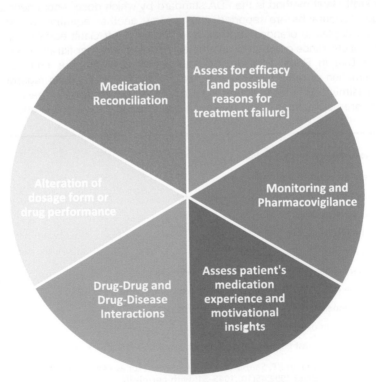

Fig. 2. Proposed checklist of polypharmacy management checklist items.

records, controlled substance refill reporting, and accounting for over-the-counter medication, supplements, herbal products, and vitamins. The process of getting accurate data is impacted by transitions of care, a patient's ability to report and keep records, clinical team time, and resources. Much of the work of medication reconciliation can be given to midlevel providers, office staff, student volunteers working in a clinic, and health care professional trainees. The data-gathering aspect can be done as much as possible before the 15-minute office visit with system implementation of medication reconciliation protocol.

The brown bag assessment means that patients bring everything they are taking at the current time in a bag to each appointment. The brown bag assessment is the gold standard for medication reconciliation (if patients remember to bring everything they are taking). The ideal is to go through the brown bag assessment at each office visit, although once per year at minimum is helpful. Sometimes patients omit some products they are taking because they do not assume, for example, that an over-the-counter medication should be part of a brown bag assessment; perhaps they perceive the brown bag should be only prescription medications. Therefore, it is important to provide a bit of training for patients to ensure that they understand they are to bring everything. Patients should also bring a list of medications they take, if they keep one, for comparison.

Medication reconciliation and initial medication use interviewing can be done by office staff, medical assistants, volunteer students, or trainees before a 15-minute office visit by going through the process of listing the contents of the bag. It is important to train whoever does the brown bag assessment to ask open-ended questions to find out if there is anything missing. Open-ended questions about how a patient is taking each medication should be recorded and compared with the instructions on the labels.

Staff or volunteers can also work to gather medication data for patients ahead of an office visit by requesting hospital discharge records, pharmacy records, and controlled substance reporting records to save time and to help ensure complete medication reconciliation during the office visit. Health Insurance Portability and Accountability Act training and credentialing for patient interaction and care are requirements before enlisting staff or volunteers to help with brown bag assessments and medication reconciliation data collection. Regarding the added time required to provide for older adult patients in the clinic setting in general, precepting students can be a bidirectionally beneficial activity. Students learn much about the complexity of patient care and gain experience, and they can be helpful to a practice setting.

Monitoring and Pharmacovigilance

- For each prescription and over-the-counter medication, consult point-of-care drug databases or the FDA drug monograph prescribing information to document, for each medication, routine laboratory studies, renal dose adjustments, top side effects, and drug-disease interactions.
- For herbal products and supplements, consult the NIH Complementary and Alternative Medicine Herbal and Natural Products Web site, where there is a list of databases that can offer resources for monitoring these products (see section on herbal products and supplements). Typically, drug interaction checkers, when including herbal, supplements, and vitamins, flag problems of product-disease or product-drug interactions accurately.

When a patient is using drugs that are new to market, a heightened approach to monitoring should be adapted. As discussed previously, clinical studies tend to exclude older adult patients, in particular frail and multimorbid patients. The exclusion of the very old and frail from safety and efficacy trials that bring drugs to market, means, expected monitoring and adverse effect recommendations for frail older adults is uncertain in new to market drugs. The case of Vioxx® (Rofecoxib) is an example of a new-to-market drug that possessed a high risk of ADEs, which was discovered through postmarketing surveillance, and a serious threat to older adults. Older adults are more susceptible to unexpected adverse outcomes with new-to-market drugs due to lack of physiologic reserve and lack of data that from postmarketing surveillance.[51]

Clinical Pearl

New-to-market medications should be avoided in older adults; older adults tend to be excluded from new drug trials, and postmarketing data typically reveal problems with medications in older adults.

Drug-Drug Interactions

At minimum, running a patient's prescription and over-the-counter medications, herbal products, and supplements through an interaction checker should be done periodically.[52] There are several available in point-of-care applications, such as Epocrates or Lexicomp, or online. Patients can be advised to help perform their own polypharmacy pharmacovigilance by running their lists through interaction checkers online, such as those found at Drugs.com or RxList. The results can then be reviewed with patients to improve self-management and medication use literacy. The patient or clinic staff could have the process of running a drug interaction checker done before the appointment with the provider. The frequency for performing interaction checkers is dependent on patients and the consistency of their total medication and product use.

Assess for Medication and Over-the-Counter Herbal or Supplement Product Efficacy

One important and commonly overlooked aspect of polypharmacy management is assessment of medication efficacy. Some medications are difficult to assess for efficacy because their effectiveness is targeted at long-term prevention, and a person's life expectancy is a variable which, therefore impacts the definition of efficacy. But, in frail older adults, when medications are used to treat a problem that affects quality of life or end-stage disease, assessment of efficacy is not as difficult to determine. One means of assessment of medication efficacy in patients treated for end-stage disease symptoms or symptoms affecting quality of life is to withhold the medication if safe to do so for a short interval to assess utility and safety of that medication's use. Two examples where discovering ineffective medication is useful in older adults are overactive bladder medications and loop diuretics used for lower extremity edema in patients with venous stasis. Both medication classes present significant risk for the frail and older patients who use them.

Overactive bladder medications can cause cognitive impairment and cardiac events as well as occasionally inducing overflow incontinence by causing increased postvoid residual. Patients often fail treatment in part because other modes of treatment besides pharmacotherapy should be used simultaneously, such as routine toileting. The etiologies are so complex that medications alone are not always the solution.[53,54] A study of 103,250 patients with mean age of 58.7 over 24 months taking medications for overactive bladder found that time to treatment failure was 159 days, with 91.7% failing to meet treatment goals.[55]

Lower extremity edema is common because of inactivity and diminished homeostatic venous capacity, and, in some cases, the chronic use of loop diuretics achieves little improvement while placing patients at increased risk of electrolyte disorders, impaired renal function, and stimulation of the renin angiotensin system and volume depletion.[56] Often, lack of further evaluation to determine the correct etiology leads to inappropriate loop diuretic use long-term without efficacy.[57,58] For those cases of loop diuretics resulting in little efficacy, management with increased movement and extremity elevation has been can be an effective alternative.

In general, aggressively applying a single pharmacologic mode can result in inefficacy in older patients because the problems older patients experience is so often multifactorial. One reason for treatment failure and inefficacy is that the multifactorial aspects to geriatric syndromes and problems are not evaluated. There are some medications that have not been shown widely effective, such as treatments for Alzheimer dementia, yet are difficult to stop because the decision about efficacy involves the beliefs of the caregivers and subjective findings.[59] Herbals, supplements, and vitamins are other examples of a category for which it is not easy to prove efficacy yet difficult to get patients to give up because of their belief and expectations. With herbals, supplements, and vitamins, the risk of unknown effects is problematic and it is worth attempting to gain patient trust to stop them if not needed. Explaining that herbals, supplements, and vitamins are not regulated as prescription and over-the-counter medications are by the FDA sometimes helps improve patient awareness.

Assess Alteration of Dosage Forms and the Impact of Food or Acid Suppression Therapy

Any patient, especially a person with swallowing difficulties, is liable to split tablets or open or crush capsules just to be able to take them. The challenge is that the practice of dosage form alteration can significantly alter the way the medications perform and lead to significant toxicity.[60] An Australian study showed that 17% of medications altered before administration had potential to cause increased toxicity, decreased efficacy, and safety or stability concerns, and the incidence of drug dosage form alteration was 46% in the high care setting, 34% in the intermediate care setting, and 2% in the low care setting.[61] Therefore, an important component of polypharmacy management is at least occasionally (perhaps once annually) asking patients if they split or crush any tablets that they are taking. These data might help identify any treatment failures, toxicities, or adverse effects.

If medication treatment failures or abnormalities are observed, assessment of the potential impact of acid suppression therapy and bariatric surgery should be considered.[62–64] Recently geriatrics practice are starting to see the first cohort of aging Roux-en-Y gastric bypass patients. They may present with nutrient deficiencies, which appear at first to be cognitive impairment of Alzheimer or other type of dementia, or sometimes with inability to get relief from pain medications as well as treatment failures. Also, it should be considered that when medications are developed, they are designed to perform under normal gastric circumstances in which the gastric pH is approximately 1.0, and chronic proton pump inhibitor use can elevate the gastric pH to over 4, which can alter the performance of some medications.[62,65,66]

The effect of combining medications with food should be evaluated for evaluation of medication efficacy and possible link to side effects, such as upset stomach and nausea. With tamsulosin [Flomax], the recommendations are to take one-half hour after the same meal each day and to not crush or chew. The presence of food, however, causes a lower plasma peak and lower bioavailability than an empty stomach (30% increase in bioavailability and up to 70% higher plasma peak), meaning that instead of increasing the dose of tamsulosin from 0.4 mg to 0.8 mg, a provider might try having the patient take it on an empty stomach in the morning, one-half hour before breakfast, to attempt to gain better efficacy, if the patient can tolerate the drug on an empty stomach.

Assess Patient Medication Use Experience and Patient-centered Medication Use Risks

There are multiple patient-centered factors that influence successful medication use and risk of medication use failures, for example, health literacy, cognitive impairment, recent transitions of care (hospitalization and rehabilitation stay), socioeconomic barriers to consistent medication access, and multiple providers. The following checklist represents patient-centered screens for medication or polypharmacy related patient-centered risks:

- Health literacy screening[67]
- Morisky scale (adherence screen)[68]
- Any recent hospitalization or transitions of care or institutionalization?
- Barrier to medication access
  - Transportation
  - Medicare D doughnut hole
  - Uncovered medications

Motivational interviewing to detect a patient's actual medication experience includes the use of open-ended questions. Ideally, going through the medication list one by one and asking what the medication is for, is it working, and if there are there any problems can be revealing. The ultimate driver of adherence is the belief that a medication works, which is strongly supported by feedback either by perceivable action or fostered by health care professional education and health literacy enforcement. Thus, medications, such as zolpidem (Ambien), which provide immediate feedback that they work, are adhered to closely. For statins, adherence is not driven as much by feedback. The discovery of subtle problems related to a patient's medication experience or common barriers, such as uncovered medications, might trigger a good time for a referral for CMM services (through Medicare D benefit or other, as discussed previously).

SUMMARY

The management of polypharmacy in a 15-minute office visit presents a significant challenge in older adults, yet the PCP and the patient-centered medical home seem to be the optimal places to implement overall medication management. Creating a systematic method to address polypharmacy in older patients, by looking to minimize the use of PIMs, performing CMR at least once annually (perhaps as part of the Medicare annual wellness visit), working with the office or extended community team (referral for CMM through Medicare D partners), and ensuring appropriate monitoring can go a long way toward improving outcomes and avoiding medication-related misadventure. Each practice has different polypharmacy management needs based on patient demographics, location, and health system parameters. Fortunately, there are growing varieties of resources online and in communities to make successful medication management a reality. Taking the time to curate a system and network for a practice will provide significant returns on investment via avoided hospitalization, increased billing levels, and heightened quality measure bonuses, but most of all, patients will feel empowered and more functional with improved medication management and avoidance of unnecessary polypharmacy.

REFERENCES

1. McCormick WC. Revised AGS Choosing Wisely((R)) list: changes to help guide older adult care conversations. J Gerontol Nurs 2015;41(5):49–50.
2. Cherry DLC, Decker SL. Population aging and the use of office-based physician services. NCHS data brief, no 41. Hyattsville (MD): National Center for Health Statistics; 2010. CDC websight.
3. Gurwitz J, Monane M, Monane S, et al. Brown University long-term care quality letter. American Society on Aging—National Council on Aging Annual Conference. 2001.
4. Van Spall HG, Toren A, Kiss A, et al. Eligibility criteria of randomized controlled trials published in high-impact general medical journals: a systematic sampling review. JAMA 2007;297(11):1233–40.
5. Tai-Seale M, McGuire T. Time is up: increasing shadow price of time in primary-care office visits. Health Econ 2012;21(4):457–76.
6. Sganga F, Landi F, Ruggiero C, et al. Polypharmacy and health outcomes among older adults discharged from hospital: results from the CRIME study. Geriatr Gerontol Int 2015;15(2):141–6.
7. Gamble JM, Hall JJ, Marrie TJ, et al. Medication transitions and polypharmacy in older adults following acute care. Ther Clin Risk Manag 2014;10:189–96.
8. Fried TR, O'Leary J, Towle V, et al. Health outcomes associated with polypharmacy in community-dwelling older adults: a systematic review. J Am Geriatr Soc 2014;62(12):2261–72.
9. Garfinkel D, Zur-Gil S, Ben-Israel J. The war against polypharmacy: a new cost-effective geriatric-palliative approach for improving drug therapy in disabled elderly people. Isr Med Assoc J 2007;9(6):430–4.
10. Hilmer SN, Mager DE, Simonsick EM, et al. A drug burden index to define the functional burden of medications in older people. Arch Intern Med 2007;167(8):781–7.
11. Hilmer SN, Gnjidic D, Abernethy DR. Drug Burden Index for international assessment of the functional burden of medications in older people. J Am Geriatr Soc 2014;62(4):791–2.
12. Jodar-Sanchez F, Malet-Larrea A, Martin JJ, et al. Cost-utility analysis of a medication review with follow-up service for older adults with polypharmacy in community pharmacies in Spain: the conSIGUE program. Pharmacoeconomics 2015; 33(6):599–610.
13. Wittayanukorn S, Westrick SC, Hansen RA, et al. Evaluation of medication therapy management services for patients with cardiovascular disease in a self-insured employer health plan. J Manag Care Pharm 2013;19(5):385–95.
14. Brummel A, Lustig A, Westrich K, et al. Best practices: improving patient outcomes and costs in an ACO through comprehensive medication therapy management. J Manag Care Spec Pharm 2014;20(12):1152–8.
15. Gazda NP, Berenbrok LA, Ferreri SP. Comparison of two Medication Therapy Management Practice Models on Return on Investment. J Pharm Pract 2016; 30(3):282–5.
16. By the American Geriatrics Society Beers Criteria Update Expert Panel. American Geriatrics Society 2015 updated beers criteria for potentially inappropriate medication use in older adults. J Am Geriatr Soc 2015;63(11):2227–46.
17. O'Mahony D, O'Sullivan D, Byrne S, et al. STOPP/START criteria for potentially inappropriate prescribing in older people: version 2. Age Ageing 2015;44(2): 213–8.

18. Cipolle RJ, Cipolle RJ, Morley PC, et al. Pharmaceutical care practice. 3rd edition. New York: McGraw-Hill; 2012.

19. Woodall T, Landis SE, Galvin SL, et al. Provision of annual wellness visits with comprehensive medication management by a clinical pharmacist practitioner. Am J Health Syst Pharm 2017;74(4):218–23.

20. Collaborative PCPC. Integrating comprehensive medicaiton management to optimize patient outcomes. 2nd edition. PCPCC Resource Guide on Integrating CMM. Washington, DC: Patient Centered Primacy Care Collaborative; 2012. Available at: https://www.pcpcc.org/sites/default/files/media/medmanagement.pdf. Accessed February 1, 2017.

21. American College of Clinical Pharmacists. Comprehensive medication management in team-based care. Washington, DC: American College of Clinical Pharmacists Brief; 2016.

22. Gurwitz JH, Field TS, Harrold LR, et al. Incidence and preventability of adverse drug events among older persons in the ambulatory setting. JAMA 2003; 289(9):1107–16.

23. Budnitz DS, Lovegrove MC, Shehab N, et al. Emergency hospitalizations for adverse drug events in older Americans. N Engl J Med 2011;365(21):2002–12.

24. Budnitz DS, Shehab N, Kegler SR, et al. Medication use leading to emergency department visits for adverse drug events in older adults. Ann Intern Med 2007;147(11):755–65.

25. Thomsen LA, Winterstein AG, Sondergaard B, et al. Systematic review of the incidence and characteristics of preventable adverse drug events in ambulatory care. Ann Pharmacother 2007;41(9):1411–26.

26. Haynes RB, Ackloo E, Sahota N, et al. Interventions for enhancing medication adherence. Cochrane Database Syst Rev 2008;(2):CD000011.

27. Garfinkel D, Mangin D. Feasibility study of a systematic approach for discontinuation of multiple medications in older adults: addressing polypharmacy. Arch Intern Med 2010;170(18):1648–54.

28. Hilmer SN, Gnjidic D, Le Couteur DG. Thinking through the medication list - appropriate prescribing and deprescribing in robust and frail older patients. Aust Fam Physician 2012;41(12):924–8.

29. UptoDate. Available at: http://www.uptodate.com/contents/drug-prescribing-for-older-adults?source=search_result&search=prescribing+Garfinkle&selectedTitle=1%7E150#H25. Accessed May 30, 2017.

30. Jordan S, Gabe M, Newson L, et al. Medication monitoring for people with dementia in care homes: the feasibility and clinical impact of nurse-led monitoring. ScientificWorldJournal 2014;2014:843621.

31. Cousins D. Current status of the monitoring of medication practice. Am J Health Syst Pharm 2009;66(5 Suppl 3):S49–56.

32. Steinman MA, Miao Y, Boscardin WJ, et al. Prescribing quality in older veterans: a multifocal approach. J Gen Intern Med 2014;29(10):1379–86.

33. Bell SP, Saraf AA. Epidemiology of multimorbidity in older adults with cardiovascular disease. Clin Geriatr Med 2016;32(2):215–26.

34. Downing NS, Shah ND, Neiman JH, et al. Participation of the elderly, women, and minorities in pivotal trials supporting 2011–2013 U.S. Food and Drug Administration approvals. Trials 2016;17(1):199.

35. Boyd CM, Vollenweider D, Puhan MA. Informing evidence-based decision-making for patients with comorbidity: availability of necessary information in clinical trials for chronic diseases. PLoS One 2012;7(8):e41601.

36. Boyd CM, Darer J, Boult C, et al. Clinical practice guidelines and quality of care for older patients with multiple comorbid diseases: implications for pay for performance. JAMA 2005;294(6):716–24.
37. Romera L, Orfila F, Segura JM, et al. Effectiveness of a primary care based multifactorial intervention to improve frailty parameters in the elderly: a randomised clinical trial: rationale and study design. BMC Geriatr 2014;14:125.
38. Yourman LC, Lee SJ, Schonberg MA, et al. Prognostic indices for older adults: a systematic review. JAMA 2012;307(2):182–92.
39. Min L, Yoon W, Mariano J, et al. The vulnerable elders-13 survey predicts 5-year functional decline and mortality outcomes in older ambulatory care patients. J Am Geriatr Soc 2009;57(11):2070–6.
40. Peron EP, Gray SL, Hanlon JT. Medication use and functional status decline in older adults: a narrative review. Am J Geriatr Pharmacother 2011;9(6):378–91.
41. Hilmer SN, Mager DE, Simonsick EM, et al. Drug burden index score and functional decline in older people. Am J Med 2009;122(12):1142–9.e1-2.
42. Hilmer SN, Gnjidic D. The effects of polypharmacy in older adults. Clin Pharmacol Ther 2009;85(1):86–8.
43. Bennett A, Gnjidic D, Gillett M, et al. Prevalence and impact of fall-risk-increasing drugs, polypharmacy, and drug-drug interactions in robust versus frail hospitalised falls patients: a prospective cohort study. Drugs Aging 2014;31(3):225–32.
44. Best O, Gnjidic D, Hilmer SN, et al. Investigating polypharmacy and drug burden index in hospitalised older people. Intern Med J 2013;43(8):912–8.
45. Funnell M. What's new in the 2013 guidelines for diabetes care? Nursing 2013; 43(7):66.
46. Nguyen V, deGoma EM, Hossain E, et al. Updated cholesterol guidelines and intensity of statin therapy. J Clin Lipidol 2015;9(3):357–9.
47. Armstrong C, Joint National Committe. JNC8 guidelines for the management of hypertension in adults. Am Fam Physician 2014;90(7):503–4.
48. Ickowicz E, American Geriatrics Society Expert Panel on the Care of Older Adults with Multimorbidity. Patient-centered care for older adults with multiple chronic conditions: a stepwise approach from the American Geriatrics Society. J Am Geriatr Soc 2012;60(10):1957–68.
49. Excellencje NBNIfHaC. Medicines Optimisation: the safe and effective use of medicienes to enable the best possible outcomes. NICE guideline NG5. 2015. Available at: https://www.nice.org.uk/guidance/service-delivery–organisation-and-staffing/medicines-management. Accessed February 1, 2017.
50. Paige NM, Nagami GT. The top 10 things nephrologists wish every primary care physician knew. Mayo Clin Proc 2009;84(2):180–6.
51. Antimisiaris D, Miles T, Leey-Casella J, et al. New medical treatments: risks and benefits in practice. Gerontologist 2008;48:303.
52. Hanlon JT, Sloane RJ, Pieper CF, et al. Association of adverse drug reactions with drug-drug and drug-disease interactions in frail older outpatients. Age Ageing 2011;40(2):274–7.
53. Chapple C. Chapter 2: pathophysiology of neurogenic detrusor overactivity and the symptom complex of "Overactive Bladder". Neurourol Urodyn 2014;33:S6–13.
54. Meng E, Lin WY, Lee WC, et al. Pathophysiology of overactive bladder. Low Urin Tract Symptoms 2012;4:48–55.
55. Chancellor MB, Migliaccio-Walle K, Bramley TJ, et al. Long-term patterns of use and treatment failure with anticholinergic agents for overactive bladder. Clin Ther 2013;35(11):1744–51.

56. Schartum-Hansen H, Loland KH, Svingen GF, et al. Use of loop diuretics is associated with increased mortality in patients with suspected coronary artery disease, but without systolic heart failure or renal impairment: an observational study using propensity score matching. PLoS One 2015;10(6):e0124611.

57. Thaler HW, Pienaar S, Wirnsberger G, et al. Bilateral leg edema in an older woman. Z Gerontol Geriatr 2015;48(1):49–51.

58. Ely JW, Osheroff JA, Chambliss ML, et al. Approach to leg edema of unclear etiology. J Am Board Fam Med 2006;19(2):148–60.

59. Casey DA, Antimisiaris D, O'Brien J. Drugs for Alzheimer's disease: are they effective? P T 2010;35(4):208–11.

60. Gopalraj RK, Antimisiaris DE, O'Brien JG, et al. Glossodynia: an unsuspected etiology. J Am Geriatr Soc 2009;57:S119.

61. Paradiso L. Crushing or altering medications: what's happening in residential aged-care facilities? Australas J Ageing 2002;21(3):123–7.

62. Ogawa R, Echizen H. Drug-drug interaction profiles of proton pump inhibitors. Clin Pharmacokinet 2010;49(8):509–33.

63. Miller AD, Smith KM. Medication use in bariatric surgery patients: what orthopedists need to know. Orthopedics 2006;29(2):121–3.

64. Miller AD, Smith KM. Medication and nutrient administration considerations after bariatric surgery. Am J Health Syst Pharm 2006;63(19):1852–7.

65. Shin JM, Sachs G. Pharmacology of proton pump inhibitors. Curr Gastroenterol Rep 2008;10(6):528–34.

66. Sachs G, Shin JM, Howden CW. Review article: the clinical pharmacology of proton pump inhibitors. Aliment Pharmacol Ther 2006;23(Suppl 2):2–8.

67. Louis AJ, Arora VM, Press VG. Evaluating the brief health literacy screen. J Gen Intern Med 2014;29(1):21.

68. Morisky DE, Ang A, Krousel-Wood M, et al. Predictive validity of a medication adherence measure in an outpatient setting. J Clin Hypertens (Greenwich) 2008;10(5):348–54.

Geriatric Assessment for Primary Care Providers

Hong-Phuc T. Tran, MD[a],[*], Susan D. Leonard, MD[b]

KEYWORDS

- Geriatric • Assessment • Function • Elder • Geriatric syndrome • Older adult

KEY POINTS

- Cognitive deficits, delirium, functional decline, falls, incontinence, pressure ulcers, and frailty are examples of geriatric syndromes.
- A comprehensive geriatric assessment evaluates multiple domains, including social, functional, economic, psychosocial, cognitive, and environmental, and uses interdisciplinary teams to develop a coordinated plan of care for the older adult.
- In the geriatric population, the initial sign of a medical problem may be a change or decline in function and mental status, rather than a clinical or laboratory abnormality.
- Assessment tools can help reduce the burden of work in performing comprehensive geriatric assessments; additionally, office staff can be trained to take larger roles in assessing and monitoring older adults.

INTRODUCTION

Because of a growing, aging population and worsening shortage of geriatricians in the United States, the care of geriatric patients will mostly devolve to primary care providers. In 2004, there was an estimated 1 fellowship-trained geriatrician for every 10,350 Americans aged 75 years and older.[1] Hence, it is imperative that primary care providers be trained and comfortable with managing geriatric syndromes and multiple chronic medical conditions, as well as delivering high-quality, cost-effective care to the elderly. In 2011, the first cohort of the American baby boomers (those born between 1945 and 1966) reached age 65 years and, by 2030, 1 in every 5 Americans will be 65 years of age and older.[1] Medicare beneficiaries with 4 or more chronic conditions generate 80% of all Medicare spending.[1] Preparing primary care physicians to provide expert geriatric chronic care and increasing the workforce of primary care physicians can help older adults receive better access to skilled providers and

This article originally appeared in *Primary Care Clinics: Clinics in Office Practice*, Volume 44, Issue 3, September 2017.

Conflicts of interest: The authors have no conflicts of interest to report.

[a] Division of Geriatrics, UCLA, 1223 16th Street, Suite 3100, Los Angeles, CA, USA; [b] Division of Geriatrics, UCLA, 200 Medical Plaza, Suite 365-A, Los Angeles, CA 90095, USA

* Corresponding author.

E-mail address: hongphuctran@mednet.ucla.edu

help improve the Medicare budgetary crisis. This article focuses on geriatric assessment for primary care providers.

MULTIFACTORIAL AND MULTIDISCIPLINARY APPROACH

The geriatric medical assessment is an important diagnostic tool to use while assessing the elderly. Older individuals may have more comorbidities and impairments that contribute to functional decline, and recognizing how various disciplines work together to affect outcome can guide decision making and medical management. The assessment goes beyond just medical conditions to include a spectrum of systems including social, functional, economic, psychosocial, cognitive, and environmental conditions.[2] Ranging from brief screens to more extensive evaluations, the geriatric assessment addresses how the domains interplay to affect functional status.

The functional evaluation is a fundamental concept in the framework of the geriatric assessment. Functional status can be seen as a measure of overall health impact in the context of an individual's environment and social support network. As individuals live longer, they survive longer with functional impairments. In the geriatric population, the initial sign of a medical problem may be a decline or change in function rather than a clinical abnormality. Effective medical management accounts for overall function instead of management of acute symptoms.

PHYSICAL HEALTH AND INTRODUCTION TO GERIATRIC SYNDROMES

When assessing the physical health of geriatric patients, different components need to be taken into account, such as acute and chronic medical issues, vision and hearing, continence, nutrition, gait, and sleep disorders.

Geriatric syndrome is a term used to describe unique health conditions in elderly patients that are multifactorial in cause and do not fit into discrete organ-based categories. Examples of geriatric syndromes include functional decline, falls, frailty, incontinence, and pressure ulcers.[3] Cognitive deficits and delirium are geriatric syndromes that are discussed elsewhere in this issue. Frailty is an impairment in mobility, balance, endurance, physical activity, muscle strength, nutrition, and cognition; it is the overarching geriatric syndrome.[3] The constellation of other geriatric syndromes (such as falls, delirium, functional decline, and/or pressure ulcers) can lead to frailty, and frailty itself can feed back to result in the development of more risk factors and, in turn, even more geriatric syndromes, with the final outcomes being disability, dependence, and death.[3]

MEDICAL

Primary care providers need to be adept at diagnosing and managing the geriatric syndromes (mentioned earlier) and common medical conditions in older adults. The geriatric assessment should be comprehensive and holistic; however, time constraints may limit the realistic ability to perform thorough evaluations. The medical assessment of older adults can be done by physicians, nurse practitioners, or physician assistants; efficiency in the office visit can be achieved by using medical assistants and/or nurses to help with data gathering and performing standardized assessments.

Older adults often present with vague complaints, such as dizziness, and may have cognitive deficits that affect their ability to provide a concise, accurate history. They may under-report or over-report symptoms. In a brief office encounter, it may be difficult to obtain all the relevant details in a timely manner. Hence, eliciting collateral information from the patient's family or caregivers can greatly help the primary care provider in making a diagnostic evaluation. For older adults with cognitive deficits who come to their appointments alone, the primary care provider can consider calling the family or caregiver to "attend" the interview portion of the visit via telephone conference. If a geriatric patient lives in an assisted-living or board-and-care facility, contacting the facility for an updated medication list and collateral information is helpful. Previsit and self-report questionnaires can also help with information gathering and can be done by trained office staff. Medication reconciliation can also be performed by office staff.

VISION AND HEARING

Sensory deficits can greatly affect the quality of life of older adults. About 16% of adults 75 to 84 years old and 27% of those 85 years of age and older are unable to read newsprint (even with correction lenses). Cataracts, age-related macular degeneration, and glaucoma are common causes of vision problems in older adults. Vision loss is a risk factor for hip fractures and motor-vehicle accidents and is associated with faster physical decline and greater mortality. Screening for (and correcting) vision loss may prevent these effects.[4] The Snellen eye chart is a quick way to assess vision.

Age-related sensorineural hearing loss is a common problem in geriatric patients, and can lead to social isolation, depression, and reduced quality of life. Presbycusis is the most common cause of hearing loss, and is the progressive decline in ability to perceive high-frequency tones, caused by degeneration of hair cells in the ear. Hearing loss is associated with falls, cognitive and physical decline, and increased mortality. The Whisper test, finger rub, or handheld audiometer can be used to assess hearing and can be done by office staff. For patients with moderate to severe hearing deficits, a pocket-talker (see https://www.hearingspeech.org/services/hearing-aids/assistive-listening-devices/) can be used to amplify sound and help patients hear, potentially making the office visit more efficient. Referrals to audiologists for further hearing evaluation and assessment for hearing aids can be made if indicated.[5]

URINARY INCONTINENCE

Urine incontinence is a common source of emotional distress and embarrassment for older adults and can lead to social isolation. Despite being common, many community-dwelling older adults with urinary incontinence, especially women, do not seek help from their medical providers.[6] The presence of urine incontinence can be assessed with brief screening questionnaires, postvoid residual (if bladder scanner is available), and urine dipstick. A postvoid residual can assist with determining whether urine retention is contributing to overflow urinary incontinence. A urine dipstick can help rule out a urinary tract infection. In older adults using multiple medications, assessment of medications and their potential contributions to urinary incontinence should be performed (for a review and resources regarding the assessment of urinary incontinence see http://www.aafp.org/afp/2013/0415/p543.html#afp20130415p543-f1). Patient resources can be found at the National Association for Continence (see https://www.nafc.org/urinary-incontinence/).

NUTRITION

Nutritional status in older adults is determined by multiple factors, such as comorbid medical conditions, activity level, energy expenditure, and caloric requirements. The ability to access, prepare, ingest, and digest food, and also appetite, are important considerations. Nutrition can be assessed by weight, height, and body mass index.

Because of decreased physiologic reserves associated with increasing age, older adults are at increased risk of malnutrition, especially after an acute illness or hospitalization. There are various criteria for clinically significant weight loss; the Centers for Medicare and Medicaid Services' Resident Assessment Instrument (RAI) Minimum Data Set (MDS) Version 3.0 uses the proposed criteria of weight loss of 5% or greater of baseline body weight in 30 days, or 10% or more of baseline body weight in 6 months for nursing facility patients (see https://www.cms.gov/Medicare/Quality-Initiatives-Patient-Assessment-Instruments/NursingHomeQualityInits/Downloads/MDS-30-RAI-Manual-V113.pdf).

For patients with significant weight loss, it is important to assess psychological, socioeconomic, and cognitive factors that may be contributing to the older patient's nutritional decline. For example, cognitive decline can lead to swallowing difficulties and depression may lead to anorexia. A social worker on the interdisciplinary team can help assess the older patient's living situation and available resources. Similarly, a psychologist on the team can help with psychotherapy and management of depression and other mood disorders. Meal delivery services, such as Meals on Wheels or local delivery programs, can help improve accessibility to food. The Area Agencies on Aging (see https://www.n4a.org/aaastitlevi) can help patients access services geared toward aging in place, and Meals on Wheels is one such service. Nutritional supplements, such as protein shakes, offered 1 to 3 times daily can help older adults gain weight. After a thorough review of the patient's medications and medical, socioeconomic, and psychological history, the medical provider can devise a plan of care that suits the needs and goals of the patient. Appetite stimulants can also be considered if indicated. Keep in mind that megestrol is listed as a Beers Criterion (see http://onlinelibrary.wiley.com/doi/10.1111/jgs.13702/pdf) potentially inappropriate medication in the elderly because it can increase risk of cardiovascular thrombi and is of controversial efficacy. Mirtazapine is also used to stimulate appetite, and that effect is typically observed with low-dose use, at which level the drug has primarily antihistaminic activity (at higher doses it has increased serotonergic activity).[7]

SLEEP

Changes in sleep are a normal part of aging; however, they can be problematic for older adults who consider good sleep important to quality of life. Common sleep complaints include difficulty falling asleep, nighttime awakening, early morning awakening, and daytime sleepiness. Risk factors associated with sleep disorders include underlying mood disorder, dementia, comorbid medical conditions, and use of multiple medications.[8,9]

Assessment of sleep in older adults should include the following elements:

- Typical bedtime and rise time on weekdays and weekends
- Presence of daily sleep routine or ritual (eg, what does the patient do before going to sleep?)
- Difficulty falling or staying asleep or both
- Presence and frequency of daytime naps and their duration
- Quality of sleep (eg, does the patient feel refreshed after waking up after a night's sleep? How many times does the patient wake up during sleep? How long does it take for patient to fall back to sleep?)
- Presence of snoring or apnea
- Presence of restless legs syndrome
- Presence of daytime drowsiness or fatigue
- Presence or absence of shift work

- Activities that are affected by poor sleep
- Use of sleep aids
- Presence of depression

Assessment of sleep disorders should also include a thorough review of the patient's medications to identify any possible causes (eg, if a patient is on diuretics, is the patient taking the diuretic in the afternoon or evening?). A sleep diary detailing these elements is helpful in assessing for the presence of a sleep disorder. The consensus sleep diary, which is a standard sleep diary developed by a panel of insomnia experts, can be given to patients to complete and can be used to assess for sleep disorders; there are 3 different versions of the consensus sleep diary (with different formatting/charts) available for medical providers to use. In a busy clinic practice, time can be saved by giving a sleep diary to patients or their families to complete and having the patient return to discuss the findings in the sleep diary and treatment recommendations.[10]

Encouraging behavioral measures, such as good sleep hygiene, is key to improving sleep. Features of good sleep hygiene include minimizing daytime naps, keeping a regular bedtime and routine of relaxation, avoiding television in bed, and minimizing excessive fluid intake a few hours before bedtime. Hypnotics (benzodiazepines, non-benzodiazepines, anticholinergics like tricyclic antidepressants, and antihistamines like diphenhydramine) should be avoided because they carry increased risk of confusion, delirium, falls, and adverse side effects.[11]

MEDICATIONS AND POLYPHARMACY

A thorough review of medication adverse side effects, drug-drug interactions, and medication adherence is crucial in determining whether medications are contributing to a patient's symptoms or functional impairment. Office staff can be trained to assist with medication reconciliation and medication refills. The topic of polypharmacy is further discussed elsewhere in this issue.

FUNCTIONAL ASSESSMENT

Activities of daily living (ADLs) are used to assess function in elderly. These are divided into 3 levels: basic activities of daily living (BADLs; commonly referred to as simply ADLs), instrumental ADLs (IADLs), and advanced ADLs (AADLs).

BADLs are self-care activities that an individual must accomplish in order to survive self-sufficiently. These activities include bathing, dressing, toileting, transferring, maintaining continence, and feeding. Patients tend to lose these abilities in this order, and regain them in the opposite order during rehabilitation. Inability to perform these tasks indicates the need for additional caregiver assistance or placement into a higher level of care.

IADLs are higher-level activities that an individual must perform or have help with in order to remain independent in their living environments. These activities include using the telephone, shopping, doing housework, doing laundry, preparing meals, driving, taking medications, and managing money. Dependency in IADLs is more common and the progressive loss of more IADL functions translates to more difficulty remaining independent in the household. Some social services are available to provide assistance with these needs, such as meal delivery and transportation services. Assisted living facilities can provide help with IADLs, but usually not for BADLs unless for an additional cost.

The clinical implications are important because ADL impairment can lead to functional decline, decreased quality of life, and loss of independence. Furthermore, it can affect prognosis and hospital outcomes, and predict morbidity and mortality.[12]

Early intervention through detection of functional decline leads to reductions in negative outcomes. Changes in functional activity can also be a stronger predictor than admitting diagnoses, and other indices of illness burden. Many older patients lose some aspect of function or independence in their ADLs after being hospitalized.[12] Some risk factors include IADL impairments before admission, advanced age, and preexisting cognitive impairment.[13,14]

AADLs are more advanced tasks require a higher level of understanding and integration into societal and community roles. Examples include occupational, recreational, and travel activities. A decline in the ability to perform such tasks is often the first sign of functional change before disability.

Furthermore, understanding baseline function provides insight into setting appropriate expectations and goals. Older adults who are hospitalized should be asked about their functional status before admission to compare with the level of function at the time of discharge. Individuals in the nursing home generally depend on their IADLs, so assessing ADL capabilities becomes more relevant.

A previsit questionnaire can be helpful in making such assessments, staying mindful that most answers are by self or proxy (informant such as caregiver, family, friend) report and may have intrinsic variability. Having such questionnaires completed in advance saves time and also provides insight into the individual's concerns and cognitive ability. The Lawton IADL and Katz ADL questionnaires (see https://clas.uiowa.edu/socialwork/sites/clas.uiowa.edu.socialwork/files/NursingHomeResource/documents/Katz%20ADL_LawtonIADL.pdf) are standard screening tools for ADL and IADLs.

Many individuals tend to over-report their abilities, whereas family members may under-report abilities. Evaluation from physical and occupational therapists can provide a more objective perspective on a person's capabilities and help guide rehabilitation goals and care needs.

Functional status is essential as a basis for following the progress of patients with chronic disabilities. The functional assessment can provide valuable prognostic information to direct appropriate diagnostic evaluation, treatment plans, and goal discussions. Changes or losses in function should be understood in a context beyond just the medical conditions, and should address the environmental and social supports that interplay to affect older people's needs and goals.

GAIT AND MOBILITY ASSESSMENT

Fall-related injuries are associated with decline in functional status, increased morbidity and mortality, and increased likelihood of nursing home placement.[15] The ability to get up after a fall and the fear of falling are associated with worse outcomes and increased risk of institutionalization.

The timed Get Up and Go test can be used to screen gait, balance, and mobility in older adults. In this test, the patient is asked to rise from a standard arm chair, walk 3 m (10 feet) across the room, turn around, walk back to the chair, and sit down. More than 16 seconds to complete this test suggest an increased risk of falling, functional decline, and poor health.[16] Time-saving measures can be achieved by having office staff perform the Get up and Go test. Gait and mobility assessment can help identify older adults who would benefit from assistive devices, such as cane or walker, and physical therapy. Gait, balance, and strengthening exercises can help minimize risk of falls in older adults. Older adults who need to be lifted or who require more than 1 person's assistance to move can rarely be accommodated in their own homes; they may need hired caregivers to remain living in their own homes or placement in assisted living facilities or nursing homes where additional support staff are available.

SOCIAL/ENVIRONMENTAL ASSESSMENT

The well-being of the elderly is greatly influenced by social conditions, more so than other age groups. Because so much of elderly health is affected by the patients' social environments and support networks, sufficient understanding of the social history is necessary to provide effective patient care. Knowing the main source of support at home may include involvement of family, friends, or outside assistance for caregiving. It is also important to recognize the individual's personal values, preferences, and goals, and (more importantly) whether these goals are realistic in the context of the patient's functional status.

The social history should involve asking about the living environment and home safety, support structure, family relationships, education, habits, caregiving needs, exercise, community involvement, and advanced care planning. Other important questions include addressing financial security, safety, and injury risk.

Understanding an elderly person's living conditions can give insight into that person's overall health status. Many seniors want to remain in their own home environment. However, the living environment may be unsafe or be a leading area of injury from falls. Falls are common in the elderly and contribute to loss of independence and increased morbidity and mortality.

Home safety evaluation can reveal many high-risk conditions and correcting these can improve the home setting. Some hazards can be quickly corrected, whereas others may require more substantial home modification or prompt changing into a different environment or higher level of care. Usually home safety evaluations can be conducted by home health from a physical or occupational therapist.

Understanding the social support and caregiving status is critical in the older population. Adequate care is necessary for safety at home. Caregivers should be screened for caregiver burnout and, if concerned, referred to support groups or work on alternative caregiving arrangements.

It is important to assess for basic habits and behaviors, including tobacco, alcohol, and substance abuse in the elderly, because these may not be obvious. Habits have an effect on health outcomes, especially those that have accumulated over decades. Mortality can be delayed even in smokers who quit after the age of 70 years. Substance abuse cessation is encouraged in the elderly.

Exercise can have numerous beneficial effects and can improve cardiovascular and cerebrovascular health, decrease pain, and improve mortality. It also improves balance, flexibility, fitness, mood, sleep, and cognition. Information on physical activity and status on a patient can help prognosticate functional outcomes.

Sexual activity and health remain relevant in the elderly. Sexually transmitted diseases and human immunodeficiency virus are increasing in the older population and it is important to ask the necessary questions. Similarly, many people are concerned about the opposite problem: sexual dysfunction. Impotence and sexual dysfunction are often not discussed easily, although they are common. It is important to obtain the relevant information in the history to discuss potential treatment options.

Furthermore, elder mistreatment is a topic that should not be overlooked. The National Research Council defines mistreatment of older adults as "intentional actions that cause harm or create a serious risk of harm (whether or not harm is intended) to a vulnerable elder by a caregiver or other person who stands in a trust relationship to the elder. This includes failure by a caregiver to satisfy the elder's basic needs or to protect the elder from harm."[17] Risk factors for mistreatment of older adults include poverty, functional disability and dependency, frailty, and cognitive impairment. Elder mistreatment should also be screened, especially if there are concerns about suspicious skin marks, contusions, trauma, ulcers, malnutrition, or poor care without explanation. In addition to physical consequences, other forms of mistreatment include psychological mistreatment, neglect, and financial exploitation. Clinicians are in a key position to evaluate and report suspected elder abuse and mistreatment. Support for interventions can include assistance from social work staff and state adult protective services (www.napsa-now.org).

RESIDENTIAL LIVING OPTIONS AND LEVELS OF CARE

- A major question that frequently arises is whether the older person is in the right living environment, which must balance respect for a person's autonomy and independence with concerns about safety.
- Older people who do not have adequate support or the ability to live in their own homes may need to consider residential long-term settings, and a range of options are available depending on needs and resources.
- Residential care communities can be divided into several categories. Independent living facilities are senior living homes in a complex that offers recreational activities but still requires the individuals to be independent with ADLs.
- Assisted living facilities (ALFs) are options for individuals who need additional assistance with ADLs but not skilled nursing care. Services provided may include administration or supervision of medications and help with personal care, usually for an additional fee. ALFs are paid for privately, although there may be limited coverage from Medicaid and waiver programs.
- Board-and-care facilities offer a house-style living environment that houses approximately 4 to 6 residents. Care is provided by aides trained in basic nursing and personal care. Board and cares are sometimes more affordable than other, higher-level care settings but are paid for privately; some allow assistance from Medicaid or the Supplemental Security Income program.
- Nursing homes, also called skilled nursing facilities, can provide both postacute and long-term care. Short-term, posthospitalization stays for skilled services (ie, physical, occupational and speech therapy, wound care, intravenous antibiotics, gastrostomy tube management) are covered by Medicare following a 3-day hospital stay. The first 20 days are covered fully and days 21 to 100 require a copay as long as there is still an ongoing skilled need. Custodial services are provided for residents who remain in the facility long term and need continued ADL assistance. These services are covered by private pay, long-term care insurance, or Medicaid.

COGNITIVE EVALUATION

The prevalence of dementia (major neurocognitive disorder) and mild cognitive impairment (minor neurocognitive disorder) increases with age. Mild dementia is often underdiagnosed without specific screening. In the busy office setting, the Mini-Cog (3-item recall and Clock Draw Test) can be used to screen for cognitive deficits in older adults with memory complaints. It can be performed by trained office staff. If the Mini-Cog returns as abnormal, further cognitive screening can be performed. Some other validated instruments for cognitive screening include the Mini Mental Status Examination, Saint Louis University Mental Status Examination, and the Montreal Cognitive Assessment.[18] Further information on Alzheimer disease can be found elsewhere in this issue.

MOOD AND MENTAL HEALTH EVALUATION

Depression is common in older adults and adversely affects quality of life, morbidity, mortality, and health care use. Suicide rates are about twice as high in the older adult population compared with the general population, with white men more than 85 years of age at the highest risk. Many older adults with depression present to the primary care office with vague somatic complaints, such as fatigue, low energy, insomnia, or cognitive complaints. The Patient Health Questionnaire 2 (PHQ-2) (see http://www.cqaimh.org/pdf/tool_phq2.pdf) is a validated instrument used to screen for depression; it can be done quickly and can be performed by trained office staff. If abnormal, the provider should proceed with the Patient Health Questionnaire-9 (PHQ-9) to further assess depression. The PHQ-9 (see http://www.med.umich.edu/1info/FHP/practiceguides/depress/phq-9.pdf) can also be used to track response to medical therapy for depressed patients. Also, the Geriatric Depression Scale is a depression assessment tool specifically for geriatric patients, and can be acquired in multiple languages (see http://web.stanford.edu/~yesavage/GDS.html), and the Cornell Scale, which is used for depression assessment in persons with dementia (see http://geropsychiatriceducation.vch.ca/docs/edu-downloads/depression/cornell_scale_depression.pdf). These screening instruments can help identify which patients would benefit from referrals to mental health professionals, periodically assess for depression, and provide quantitative documentation of response to treatment.

PROGNOSIS AND PATIENT GOALS/ADVANCE CARE PLANNING

A follow-up concept of importance is prognosis, specifically life expectancy, if such predictors can influence the medical evaluation, management approach, and goals. Many of the decisions are guided by the patient's goals, whether it is to optimize function, prolong survival, or maximize comfort.

Advance care planning is the process by which patients and their physicians discuss the future goals of care and care preferences at the end of life. It is important to discuss these topics in a relaxed and rational environment to ensure that the decisions made reflect the type of care the individual desires. An advance directive is a legal document that comes into effect only for patients who are incapacitated and unable to speak for themselves. It allows individuals to express their wishes as well as designate a health care proxy or durable power of attorney. The older population is heterogeneous in end-of-life care preferences, and some desire comfort-oriented goals, whereas others want all treatments to prolong life regardless of condition.[19,20]

Understanding the patient's preferred goals of care may be helpful in framing treatment decisions through a shared decision-making process. Furthermore, physicians should recognize that older patients have fewer years remaining, so prognosis can be used to frame discussions about treatment options, disease prevention, and other long-term strategies. Recently many states have enacted the Medical Orders for Scope of Treatment (MOST) and Physicians Orders for Life Sustaining Treatment (POLST) forms (see http://polst.org/about/), which allow patients to have significant disease burden, in collaboration with their physicians, to document specific treatment decisions considering the patients values, alternative treatments, and goals of care, and the document becomes physicians orders. MOST and POLST forms, as well as all advance directives, should be reviewed periodically because of the changing nature of disease and functional impairment progression.

PRACTICAL APPROACH IN THE OFFICE

Clinicians understand the time constraints involved in a clinic visit and the challenges of performing a comprehensive assessment. Assessment tools and shortcuts can help reduce the burden of work in performing the initial assessment. Strategies for teamwork and cooperation with other disciplines can help make the work comprehensive but efficient. However, having an interdisciplinary assessment team is impractical in most office settings in a limited time period. Sometimes, directed and focused examinations are done when complaints can be prioritized. Also, it is wise to reevaluate

1. With whom do you live?
Please check all that apply

☐ Alone
☐ Spouse or partner
☐ Child
☐ Other family member (specify): _____
☐ Others, not family (specify): _____

2. Which of the following best describes your residence?

☐ Single-family house
☐ Condo
☐ Apartment
☐ Board & care/assisted living
☐ Nursing home
☐ Other (specify): _____

3. If living at a facility, please list name of person and the contact number for medical treatment orders:

Name: _____
Phone number: ( )

4. You are presently:

☐ Single/never married
☐ Married
☐ Divorced/separated
☐ Widowed
☐ Living with significant other

5. How many children do you have?

Number: _____

Are you in regular contact with your children? ☐ Yes ☐ No

6. How much school did you complete?

☐ Less than 8th grade
☐ Some high school
☐ High school graduate
☐ Some college
☐ College graduate
☐ Graduate school

7. You are presently (check one):

☐ Retired/not working
☐ Working part-time
☐ Working full-time

8. List your principal occupation and any other significant past occupations.

1. _____
2. _____
3. _____
4. _____
5. _____

Who would you call if you were sick and needed help? (Check all that apply)
☐ Spouse/partner ☐ Son ☐ Daughter ☐ Friend ☐ Neighbor
☐ Other (specify): _____

A. Please list name(s) and phone number(s):
Name: _____ Phone number: ( )
Name: _____ Phone number: ( )
Name: _____ Phone number: ( )

B. Do we have your permission to speak to the person(s) listed above on your behalf? ☐ Yes ☐ No

Do you employ someone to provide health related care or help you in your home? ☐ Yes ☐ No

If yes, please indicate the number of hours per day and days per week your paid helper is available to you.

Hours per day	Days per week
List number of hours:	☐ 1 ☐ 2 ☐ 3 ☐ 4 ☐ 5 ☐ 6 ☐ 7

Is this sufficient to meet your needs? ☐ Yes ☐ No

Do you get help from family members or friends in your home?
☐ Yes ☐ No

If yes, please indicate the number of hours per day and days per week your family member(s) or friend(s) are available to you.

Hours per day	Days per week
List number of hours:	☐ 1 ☐ 2 ☐ 3 ☐ 4 ☐ 5 ☐ 6 ☐ 7

Is this sufficient to meet your needs? ☐ Yes ☐ No

Do you provide care for a family member? ☐ Yes ☐ No

Do you drink alcohol, including beer and wine, or other alcohol (such as vodka, whiskey, gin)?

☐ Daily
☐ A few days a week (specify number of days: ____)
☐ Less than once a week
☐ Never

A. How much do you drink at a time? (One drink = 12 oz of beer or 8-9 oz of malt liquor or 5 oz of table wine or 1.5 oz of hard alcohol)

☐ 1 drink
☐ 2 drinks
☐ 3 drinks
☐ 4 drinks
☐ 5 or more drinks (number: ____)

B. Has anyone ever been concerned about your drinking? ☐ Yes ☐ No

Have you ever smoked cigarettes? ☐ Yes ☐ No

If yes:
Do you currently smoke cigarettes?
☐ Yes...If yes, how many packs per day? ☐ ¼ ☐ ½ ☐ 1 ☐ 1½ ☐ 2+
☐ No...If no, when did you quit? Year: _____
For how many years did you smoke? Number of years: _____
How many packs per day? ☐ ¼ ☐ ½ ☐ 1 ☐ 1½ ☐ 2+

Fig. 1. Previsit questionnaire: social history. (*From* Division of Geriatric Medicine. UCLA Healthcare. Pre-Visit Questionnaire. Copyright ©2016 The Regents of the University of California; with permission.)

Table 1
Previsit questionnaire: daily activities

Task	No Help Needed	Help Needed	Who Helps?
Feeding yourself			
Getting from bed to chair			
Getting to the toilet			
Getting dressed			
Bathing or showering			
Walking across the room (includes using cane or walker)			
Using the telephone			
Taking your medicines			
Preparing meals			
Managing money (like keeping track of expenses or paying bills)			
Moderately strenuous housework, such as doing the laundry			
Shopping for personal items like toiletries or medicines			
Shopping for groceries			
Driving			
Climbing a flight of stairs			
Getting to places beyond walking distance (eg, by bus, taxi, or car)			

From Division of Geriatric Medicine. UCLA Healthcare. Pre-Visit Questionnaire. Copyright ©2016 The Regents of the University of California; with permission.

certain parts of the geriatrics assessment (ie, assessing ADLs, falls, social history, mood, cognition), especially after hospitalization or major illnesses.

A previsit questionnaire can be time saving and help gather relevant information before the first visit. The questionnaire includes information about the medical history but also elaborates on elements of social history, including function, falls, incontinence, social supports, mood, vision/hearing, and advanced care planning (**Fig. 1, Table 1**).[21] New approaches focus on using existing office staff to help with the work flow.

With training, staff can assist with performing some assessments to save the provider time: (ie, vision and hearing, medication reconciliation, falls risk, urinary incontinence, cognitive and depression screening).

Furthermore, brief huddles before a patient session, in which the patient on the schedule is discussed, important information is alerted, and available results are provided, can facilitate a smoother work flow and maximize time efficiency.

SUMMARY

A comprehensive geriatric assessment is a multidisciplinary approach to identify medical, functional, cognitive, psychological, and socioeconomic issues in older adults. Interdisciplinary teams, consisting of the medical provider, nursing/office staff, social worker, psychologist, and others, are instrumental in developing coordinated plans of care for geriatric patients. The geriatric assessment helps determine the functional status of older adults, and can be used to determine an appropriate, safe living situation. Office staff can be trained to administer screening tools, gather data, and take on larger roles in assessing older adults to help reduce the burden of work on primary care providers.

REFERENCES

1. Boult C, Counsell S, Leipzig R, et al. The urgency of preparing primary care physicians to care for older people with chronic illness. Health Aff 2010;29(5):811–8.
2. Rosen SL, Reuben DB. Geriatric assessment tools. Mt Sinai J Med 2011;78:489.
3. Inouye S, Studenski S, Tinetti ME, et al. Geriatric syndromes: clinical, research and policy implications of a core geriatric concept. J Am Geriatr Soc 2007; 55(5):780–91.
4. Kass MA, Heuer DK, Higginbotham EJ, et al. The Ocular Hypertension Treatment Study: a randomized trial determines that topical ocular hypotensive medication delays or prevents the onset of primary open-angle glaucoma. Arch Ophthalmol 2002;120(6):701–13.
5. US Preventive Services Task Force. The guide to clinical preventive services 2014. Agency for Health Care Research and Quality; 2012.
6. Roberts RO, Jacobsen SJ, Rhodes T, et al. Urinary incontinence in a community-based cohort: prevalence and health-care seeking. J Am Geriatr Soc 1998;46(4): 467–72.
7. Laimer M, Kramer-Reinstadler K, Rauchenzauner M, et al. Effect of mirtazapine treatment on body composition and metabolism. J Clin Psychiatry 2006;67: 421–4.
8. Bloom HG, Ahmed I, Alessi CA, et al. Evidence-based recommendations for the assessment and management of sleep disorders in older persons. J Am Geriatr Soc 2009;57(5):761–89.
9. Alessi CA, Martin JL, Webber AP, et al. Randomized, controlled trial of a nonpharmacologic intervention to improve abnormal sleep/wake patterns in nursing home residents. J Am Geriatr Soc 2005;53(5):803–10.
10. Carney CE, Buysse DJ, Ancoli-Israel S, et al. The consensus sleep diary: standardizing prospective sleep self-monitoring. Sleep 2012;35(2):287–302.
11. Schroeck J, Ford J, Conway E, et al. Review of safety and efficacy of sleep medicines in older adults. Clin Ther 2016;38:2340–72.
12. Gill TM, Robison JT, Tinetti ME. Difficulty and dependence: two components of the disability continuum among community-living older persons. Ann Intern Med 1998;128:96.
13. Inouye SK, Peduzzi PN, Robison JT, et al. Importance of functional measures in predicting mortality among older hospitalized patients. JAMA 1998;279:1187.
14. Reuben DB, Solomon DH. Assessment in geriatrics. Of caveats and names. J Am Geriatr Soc 1989;37:570.
15. Tinetti ME, Williams CS. Falls, injuries due to falls, and the risk of admission to a nursing home. N Engl J Med 1997;337(18):1279–84.
16. Okumiya K, Matsubayashi K, Nakamura T, et al. The timed "up & go" test is a useful predictor of falls in community-swelling older people. J Am Geriatr Soc 1998; 46(7):928–30.
17. National Institute of Justice. Available at: https://www.nij.gov/topics/crime/elder-abuse/pages/welcome.aspx. Accessed April 27, 2017.

18. Lin JS, O'Connor E, Rossom RC, et al. Screening for cognitive impairment in older adults: a systematic review for the U.S. Preventative Services Task Force. Ann Intern Med 2013;159(9):601–12.
19. Keeler E, Guralnik JM, Tian H, et al. The impact of functional status on life expectancy in older persons. J Gerontol A Biol Sci Med Sci 2010;65:727.
20. Reuben DB, Tinetti ME. Goal-oriented patient care–an alternative health outcomes paradigm. N Engl J Med 2012;366:777.
21. Reuben DB, Leonard SD. Office-based assessment of the older adult. UptoDate; 2016. Available at: http://www.uptodate.com/contents/office-based-assessment-of-the-older-adult.

Moving?

Make sure your subscription moves with you!

To notify us of your new address, find your **Clinics Account Number** (located on your mailing label above your name), and contact customer service at:

Email: journalscustomerservice-usa@elsevier.com

800-654-2452 (subscribers in the U.S. & Canada)
314-447-8871 (subscribers outside of the U.S. & Canada)

Fax number: 314-447-8029

Elsevier Health Sciences Division
Subscription Customer Service
3251 Riverport Lane
Maryland Heights, MO 63043

*To ensure uninterrupted delivery of your subscription, please notify us at least 4 weeks in advance of move.